FINISHING
OUR
STORY

FINISHING OUR STORY

Preparing for the End of Life

GREGORY L. EASTWOOD, MD

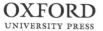

OXFORD
UNIVERSITY PRESS

OXFORD
UNIVERSITY PRESS

Oxford University Press is a department of the University of Oxford. It furthers
the University's objective of excellence in research, scholarship, and education
by publishing worldwide. Oxford is a registered trade mark of Oxford University
Press in the UK and certain other countries.

Published in the United States of America by Oxford University Press
198 Madison Avenue, New York, NY 10016, United States of America.

© Oxford University Press 2019

Library of Congress Cataloging-in-Publication Data
Names: Eastwood, Gregory L., author.
Title: Finishing our story : preparing for the end of life / Gregory L. Eastwood.
Description: New York, NY : Oxford University Press, 2019. |
Includes bibliographical references and index.
Identifiers: LCCN 2018031071 (print) | LCCN 2018045637 (ebook) |
ISBN 9780190888091 (updf) | ISBN 9780190888107 (epub) |
ISBN 9780190888084 (paperback)
Subjects: LCSH: Terminal care—Moral and ethical aspects. |
Death—Moral and ethical aspects. | BISAC: MEDICAL / Geriatrics. |
MEDICAL / Ethics. Classification: LCC R726.8 (ebook) |
LCC R726.8.E27 2019 (print) | DDC 616.02/9—dc23
LC record available at https://lccn.loc.gov/2018031071

9 8 7 6 5 4 3 2 1

Printed by Webcom Inc., Canada

To Lynn, Kristen, Lauren, Kara

CONTENTS

ACKNOWLEDGMENTS

I am grateful to Lucy Randall, my editor at Oxford University Press, for her skillful balance of flexibility and firmness and her patient management of the manuscript as well as of me throughout the process of improving it for publication. My wife, Lynn Eastwood, who understands my motivations and is an expert on my quirks, added important reality testing of the manuscript. Nancy L. Zimpher, PhD, former Chancellor of the State University of New York, saw to it that I had some sabbatical time to begin writing the book, which I very much appreciate. Kathy Faber-Langendoen, MD, Medical Alumni Endowed Professor of Bioethics and Chair of the Center for Bioethics and Humanities at SUNY Upstate Medical University, has created an extraordinary environment for professional growth and collegial enrichment, from which I have benefited. In the Center, I am surrounded by wonderful colleagues who have helped me enormously to expand my understandings of bioethics, the humanities, and medicine and health. Finally, I am indebted to all the students over my professional lifetime who have taught me a great deal and to the many patients, their families, and their doctors, nurses, social workers, and other professionals who have enriched my experiences and populated the stories that I carry in my memory and that made possible the writing of this book.

FINISHING OUR STORY

INTRODUCTION

My grandmother died when I was three years old. I made the ten-hour car trip with my parents from our home in Michigan to Yeagertown, a small town in the mountains of Pennsylvania, where my grandparents lived. I recall nothing of the trip or of the events in Yeagertown, except one thing, and it is my first memory. I am standing, holding my father's hand, in the front room of my grandparents' home, looking at Grandma lying there. Grandpa, my grandparents' children—my father and his sisters—and grandchildren and relatives and friends, all were present. Grandma was in her mid-seventies and had died from a stroke. From the perspective of decades later, I think she had what we call in the current idiom "a good death." After her stroke, her death seems to have been anticipated as being imminent and she was in the company of family and friends. She was not hospitalized, there was no diagnostic or therapeutic machinery involved, and the funeral director's fees were modest. Her minister and the church were down the street.

I wrote this book because I think many people are confused and a little put off by the end of life as it is experienced in contemporary America and many parts of the world. The experiences of the end of life and of dying, for the person who dies and for loved ones and friends, have become very different for most people from those associated with the death of my grandmother. The end of life has changed a great deal in recent years and, of course, the changes have been accompanied by enormous benefits, even regarded at times as "miracles." But sometimes they also are associated with distress, uncertainty, and conflict. This book is intended to help you understand this important part of your life and prepare for it more deliberately. You may want to ensure that the last part of your life aligns with how you have lived until then or you may want to make some adjustments that differ from how you have lived. Either way, I wish for you more control over the end of your life so as to achieve a more satisfying resolution, for you and for those who matter to you.

To most of us, the end of life and dying may be familiar in ways we do not fully comprehend. Nearly everyone knows a relative or a friend who has died and thus may appreciate some of the issues that have arisen as end of life and dying have changed. Of course, all of us will have first-hand knowledge of the end of our own lives; some readers may be experiencing that right now. And in recent years books, articles, television programs, discussion groups, and the like have opened this important part of life to better understanding and acceptance. Yet we seem to feel more at ease with, and consequently understand better, the other phases of our life—before we are born, our infancy and child-hood, and the stages of our adult years. We seem less comfortable when we anticipate the end of life. Perhaps this is related to our fears about that phase of life, avoidance of the unknown, and awareness of the finality of death.

So, this book is for people who have questions about the end of life—what to expect, how to prepare for it, what to do when you get there. I think this includes almost everybody. This view derives from my involvement in caring for patients; working as an ethics consultant, which includes interacting with patients, their families, physicians, and other health professionals; teaching end-of-life issues to medical and other health profession students; and presenting and discussing end-of-life issues with non-medical audiences.

My intention is to offer, in straightforward language, relevant information, and sometimes my own perspective, about matters that are pertinent to preparing for the process of dying—how dying has changed and why that is important, what we mean by quality of life and how that relates to end-of-life decisions, what are the implications of making one's wishes known and how to ensure that they are followed, how ethical conflicts that arise in the care of dying patients may be resolved, what palliative care is and when one might consider receiving its benefits, the facts about physician-assisted death and other forms of suicide when dying seems inevitably soon, and what it means to create the final chapter of the narrative of one's own life. To the extent that this is useful, I will be pleased.

THE BEGINNING
OF THE END

Bill stepped into the warm shower. He was pleasantly sweaty. He had fixed the garage door that morning and stacked firewood in the afternoon. Not bad for a 72-year-old guy. The diabetes was under control, and that scare about prostate cancer last year seemed to have been resolved by the surgery. He worried a little about the pain in his lower back that had developed recently and seemed to be getting worse. Today's exertions did not help that. He wondered what the MRI he had several days ago would show.

What happened next was so sudden that he had no time to process it. With a rush of rapidly fading consciousness, he lurched out of the shower and collapsed on the floor. Sue heard the thump and rushed into the bathroom. Bill was unresponsive. She took his pulse, could not detect one, and called 9-1-1. Sue turned Bill on his back and tried to compress his chest to help Bill's heart keep his blood flowing. Ten minutes later the EMTs arrived. The EMTs attached the monitor paddles—ventricular fibrillation. A couple shocks were sufficient to restore a normal heart rhythm. Bill remained unconscious as the EMTs took him to the hospital.

In the intensive care unit, Dr. Flint said to Sue, "Your husband seems to be medically stable, which is good. But the circulation to his brain was interrupted for several minutes after that episode in the shower and that concerns me."

"What do you mean?" asked Sue.

"I think that Bill may have suffered some damage to his brain. We will be better able to tell what the outlook will be in several days. It is good that his heart is back to a normal rhythm." Dr. Flint continued, "We will need to make some decisions about your husband's medical care over the next several days. Clearly, he cannot make those decisions himself and someone will need to make them for him. Does your husband have a health care proxy? A health care proxy is a person he has designated to make medical decisions for him when he is not able to make decisions for himself."

"No, I'm afraid not. We did not talk much about those things," said Sue.

"Are you willing to do that? You, as his wife, in the absence of a health care proxy, would be the person to make decisions for him, if you are willing."

Sue agreed, but she did not fully understand what she had agreed to.

Dr. Flint added, "Bill is having some trouble breathing, and we may need to pass a tube into his lungs, an endotracheal tube. That is a tube that goes through his mouth to the back of the throat and into his trachea. We would like to connect it to a ventilator, a machine that will help him breathe. Would that be OK?"

"Yes, of course, doctor. You should do whatever you need to do," said Sue.

The next day Dr. Flint told Sue that Bill was tolerating the ventilator, but he remained unconscious and his kidneys were failing, perhaps related to his diabetes and aggravated by the poor circulation when he collapsed.

"We will keep a close watch on that," said Dr. Flint. "Also, this morning I received the report of your husband's MRI of his back from your primary care doctor, and it shows something in the spine that might be related to his prostate cancer. I am sorry, but it is possible that the cancer has spread to his spine. That could explain his back pain. We will not be able to look into that problem now. We will need to wait to see how he does over the next several days."

"Also, in situations like this," added Dr. Flint, "we often ask whether the person would want a DNR order. DNR means do not resuscitate. When someone's heart stops and we try to resuscitate it, we may do several things. We press on the chest, which compresses the heart, to keep blood flowing. You did that after Bill collapsed and so did the EMTs. We also may shock the patient to try to correct an abnormal rhythm. The EMTs did that, too. Sometimes we inject medications to stimulate the heart and control blood pressure." Dr. Flint paused. "Do you think your husband would want to be resuscitated if his heart stops again or would he want a DNR order and not be resuscitated?"

"I'm not sure," said Sue. "This has all come on so suddenly. I need to think about it. Our daughter Megan is flying in from Seattle this afternoon and our son Fred is driving from Cleveland. After they arrive, we'll talk about this and get back to you. Can we see you this evening?"

"Yes, I'll be here. Would 7 o'clock be OK?" said Dr. Flint. "I think it is a good idea to talk with your children. We all should try to do what we think Bill would want. I mean, if Bill were able to tell us now, what do you think he would say about this?"

When Megan and Fred arrived, they went with Sue to see their father. Sue expanded on the situation she had described to them by phone, and they spoke with the nurses to learn the latest information. It did not look good. Bill was unable to breathe without the assistance of the ventilator, was making very little urine, and showed no evidence of recognizing or responding to Sue or Megan or Fred. They talked about the DNR order.

"Dad always was so vigorous and forward-looking," said Megan. "He would want us to try everything. He would not want them to just let him die without trying to revive his heart. Look what happened already. Mom started chest compressions and the EMTs got his heart beating again."

"I agree," said Fred. "But, I wonder if this is the beginning of the end. The prostate cancer seems to have spread to his back, and the doctors say he may not regain his ability to think or speak because his brain was without oxygen for so long. But I think it is too early now to tell."

They all agreed that Bill would not want a DNR order at this time and told that to Dr. Flint that evening.

Thus begins a story, which, in its specifics—the people involved, their hopes and values and beliefs, the diseases and disorders, and the duration and complications of them—will be unique to every person but also will resemble the stories of many others. In many stories, loved ones agree on what should be done or not done, although the decisions are difficult and uncomfortable. In other stories, loved ones disagree among themselves. Sometimes they disagree with the medical doctors and nurses. In all situations, how does the affected person and those close to him or her manage the important decisions that need to be made at the end of life? Who will make those decisions and on what basis? What are the roles of medical professionals, perhaps clergy, friends, and others? How do we prepare for this?

In the pages that follow you will learn more about how to understand and prepare for one of the most important times of your life, the end of it. We will talk about how the process of dying has changed over the past several decades and what that might mean to you. I will ask you to examine what the quality of your life means to you and how that might influence your decisions at the end of life. You will think about how you can make your wishes known to others in advance and select a person—a health care proxy agent—so that person would be able to represent your wishes if you cannot speak for yourself. We will discuss what you or your loved ones might do to help resolve conflicts among family and friends, or with medical professionals, about your care. You will consider palliative care—a different kind of care, not a cessation of care—and what role that might have at the end of your life. We will try to clarify your options if you want to end your life yourself. Finally, because each of us is the author of the story of our own life, we will see whether we can finish the last chapter of our story in the manner we would want it to end.

Chapter 1
DYING ISN'T WHAT IT USED TO BE

Nearly everything about dying is different than it was two or three generations ago. Not death itself, of course. That remains the same. But the process of dying, what happens during those days, months, even years before we die, has changed a great deal, and it can be confusing and frightening.

In the United States and many other parts of the world, we are likely to live longer than our grandparents did, we are less likely to die at home, we die for different reasons, and our dying costs more. Moreover, many of us will die after having received treatments that were unusual or unheard of generations ago, such as potent drugs to sustain blood pressure, a tube in our trachea connected to a ventilator, or kidney dialysis. Some of us experience a "social death" weeks, months, even years before biological death occurs. Antibiotics, mechanical ventilation, artificial feeding, drugs to maintain blood pressure and cardiac function, and other means of sustaining or prolonging life have become routine. Further, whereas most people died in their own homes in the past, now less than a quarter die at home, over half die in a hospital, and less than a quarter in nursing homes.[1] Dying at home used to be attended with little fuss and expense. Now end-of-life care accounts for over 10% of all health care spending and about a quarter of the Medicare budget is spent on beneficiaries in their last year of life.[2-4]

These changes in how and when we die raise questions that are common now, but probably would have seemed strange and confusing to people two or three generations ago. Should my life be extended at all costs—financial, social, and emotional? What is quality of life and how much does it matter to me? Who can make decisions about my life and health care if I am unable to make those decisions? Can I control aspects of my dying, such as whether I am resuscitated if my heart stops (DNR, Do Not Resuscitate orders), whether I have a breathing tube or mechanical respiration (DNI, Do Not Intubate orders), or even whether I may die at home? Should I choose to kill myself under certain circumstances, such as is legally permissible in the states of Oregon, Washington, Montana, Vermont, California, Colorado, and Hawaii, the District of Columbia, and several European countries? Should the costs at the end of life be controlled so that resources may be applied to other needs?

WE LIVE LONGER . . . OR A LARGER PORTION OF WHAT MIGHT HAVE BEEN

In an earlier time, death in childhood or young adulthood was common. The poet William Wordsworth captures the familiarity and acceptance of death in childhood in his poem "We Are Seven." A little girl, one of seven children, two of whom have died, replies to a visitor,

> "Two of us in the church-yard lie,
> My sister and my brother;
> And, in the church-yard cottage, I
> Dwell near them with my mother."
>
> . . .
>
> "How many are you, then," said I,
> "If they two are in heaven?"
> Quick was the little Maid's reply,
> "O Master! we are seven."
> "But they are dead; those two are dead!
> Their spirits are in heaven!"
> 'Twas throwing words away; for still
> The little Maid would have her will,
> And said, "Nay, we are seven!"

Death, always tragic, seemed more familiar. Parents had more children, some of whom might not live beyond early childhood, and mothers died more frequently in childbirth. A person could become ill at any age, often from an infectious disease, and die suddenly, sometimes without doctors knowing why. Wolfgang Amadeus Mozart died at age 35, George Gordon Lord Byron at 36, John Keats, 25. Benjamin Franklin, who lived until age 84, and Florence Nightingale, age 90, were exceptions.

The life expectancy of a baby born in 1900 in the United States was 49 years. By 1950 it had risen to about 68 years, and in 2019 it is about 80 years. Life expectancy is a statistical concept. It represents the median number of years a person is expected to live from a particular age, say, at birth, or at 50 years, or at 80 years. Median means that half of the people in a group actually will live more than the median number of years and half will die before that. In common parlance, you have a 50–50 chance of living that long. When we say that people are living longer now, we mean that the chances of living longer have improved, that the 50–50 chance is centered around a higher age, and thus life expectancy has crept up.

Gains in longevity during the first part of the twentieth century can be attributed mainly to the eradication and control of infectious diseases, especially among children. This was due largely to public health improvements: cleaner water and better disposal of sewage. The advent of antibiotics, sulfa drugs in the 1930s and penicillin in the 1940s, contributed. The development and wide use of vaccines reduced the occurrence of deadly infectious diseases, such as smallpox and polio, and further increased the likelihood of survival beyond childhood and young adulthood. Since then, prevention and control of adult diseases, especially heart disease and cerebrovascular disease, have accounted for further gains in life expectancy. The "miracles" of modern medicine, such as advanced antibiotics, better treatment of blood pressure and diabetes, cardiac surgery, improvements in the treatment of cancers, and so on, have helped.

Women have a longer life expectancy than men. A girl born in the United States now can expect, on average, to live to age 82; a boy, 77 years. The longer you live, of course, the more you have bettered the odds. While some in your birth cohort have died, you have kept on going, so your median life expectancy rises. A 50-year-old man in the United States today may expect to live another 30 years; a woman, another 33 years. If you reach 80, you have a 50–50 chance of living to about 88 or 89. This is the stuff of life insurance actuarial tables and Social Security calculations.

Average life expectancy in the United States is adversely affected by several conditions in addition to being male. Ethnic minority and lower socioeconomic status also are associated with shorter lives. Life expectancy of black women is less than that of white women by about three years. White men outlive black men by about four years. Similarly, it is disadvantageous to be poor and less well educated. This seems to be for several reasons. More affluent and better educated people are likely to have health insurance, have easier access to health care, and take advantage of established and new forms of treatment, whereas poorer and less educated people tend to be underinsured or lack insurance, have less access to health care, be more overweight, smoke cigarettes, live in unsafe neighborhoods, and eat unhealthy food.

The income gap between rich and poor is growing.[5] However, a recent study indicates that the association between life expectancy and income varies from city to city.[6] In some cities, such as New York and Los Angeles, the poor have experienced a rising life expectancy that approaches that of the middle class in those cities. In other cities, such as Detroit and Indianapolis, the difference in life expectancy between poor and more affluent seems to be widening. Why is this? Perhaps the usual reasons to which shorter life expectancy in poor people have been attributed—higher rates of smoking and being overweight, less exercise, less access to health care—are mitigated by some of the conditions of locale. For example, the coastal cities of Los Angeles and New York are less polluted than inland cities. Also, the health policies of a city, such as the ban on trans-fat and the anti-tobacco initiatives in New York, affect both rich and poor. Just as the public health measures of clean water and improved sanitation over one hundred years ago played an important role in reducing premature deaths and extending life expectancy, public health again may be key to improving health across economic classes.

A disturbing apparent reversal of the historical slow improvement in life expectancy for white middle-aged Americans has occurred recently.[7] Annual death rates have been rising in this ethnic and age group rather than falling, compared to other ethnic and age groups, and compared to counterparts in other wealthy countries. The effect is most noticeable in people with a high-school education or less. The rising death rates in this subset of middle-aged white Americans have been attributed to an increase in suicides, the so-called opioid epidemic, alcohol and substance abuse, and other consequences of poor health. Statistically, the increase in death rate and thus lower life expectancy are sufficient to adversely affect the entire group of middle-aged white Americans.

How does life expectancy at birth in the United States, one of the most medically advanced countries in the world, compare with life expectancy in other countries? Not well. According to recent estimates in the Central Intelligence Agency World Factbook,[8] the United States is down in 42nd place, with a life expectancy of 80 years. Monaco is first, enjoying an overall life expectancy of nearly 90 years, followed by Singapore and Japan, both 85 years. Canada, the United States' immediate neighbor, ranks number 21 (82 years) and the United Kingdom is number 35 (81 years). Most European nations rank above the United States. Chad is last of 224 countries with a life expectancy of 50 years. The poor showing of the United States compared with most other developed countries is attributed to the blended effects of the wide variability in health care and health outcomes in the United States. People who have access to good health care in the United States seem to do about as well as those in countries with longer life expectancies, but that privilege is not enjoyed by everyone in the United States.

I said earlier that the longer you live, the more your median life expectancy rises. But clearly this does not go on forever. The longer we live, the prospects of living longer become slimmer and slimmer as we approach death, and we eventually die. Why is that? Simply, we are programmed to die. The program is written in our genetic code and governs the development and aging process throughout our entire life, from conception to death. These genetic instructions play out in our cells, which in turn affect our organs, and finally disable the alliance of our organs that constitutes our bodies. One or another organ deteriorates and does not work and eventually the system calls it quits and we die. Of course, contemporary medicine is all about treating dysfunction, preserving function, and delaying the inevitable, and we hope that that can be done without too much compromise in what we regard as the quality of our life. But as we consider, in the next chapter, what quality of life means to each of us, we will acknowledge that everyone experiences the inexorable descent from what we have come to accept as our normal abilities to think and act and control our bodies.

To delay or modify this inevitable process has been a preoccupation of humankind forever, and the wish to reverse the aging process has spawned the Faust legends, searches for the Fountain of Youth, and, less poetically, an abundance of multimillion-dollar industries offering creams, cosmetics, clothes, and plastic surgery. Ah! To be young again! If I can't do that, perhaps I can ameliorate the aging process and delay my death. To a limited extent this is realistic, through healthy living habits and sometimes through medical interventions, and who knows what the future may bring, but it is safe to say that dying and aging will remain intrinsic to the human condition for a long time.

DO YOU WANT TO LIVE FOREVER? OR PERHAPS JUST 200 OR 300 YEARS?

How long would it be possible for us to live if our genetics, health, and good luck all were aligned? This question raises the notion of maximum possible duration of life or potential lifespan. The maximum possible duration of life of some individuals within the human species seems to be about 110 to 120 years, meaning that some world record holders have lived upward of 120 years, but no one lives 150 years. So when we talk about increasing life expectancy, we are not talking about increasing the potential lifespan, but rather capturing a greater portion of what might have been. Conversely, when we say that someone has died prematurely, implicitly we acknowledge that the person should have lived more of his or her potential lifespan.

Another way of living longer would be to extend the limits of human life, which are controlled by our genetic program, and thus lengthen our potential lifespan. It seems likely that may happen soon because of recent research in manipulating the genetic code to change the genes that control the aging process and lead to death. The prospect of making death "optional" has attracted the attention of investors who see the economic payoffs associated with the interests of people living longer.[9] And even the prestigious National Academy of Medicine, through its Grand Challenge in Healthy Longevity, is offering $25,000,000 for breakthroughs that will extend life. Further, scientists at Case Western Reserve University have identified a molecular pathway, presumably under genetic control, that affects lifespan and health in worms and mice. They reported that increasing the tissue levels of certain proteins called Kruppel-like transcription factors produced worms and mice that lived longer and healthier lives.[10] First worms and mice, next people!

Let's speculate on what might happen if humankind does develop the ability to delay death, say, to 150 or 200 years of age. Is that what we want? Do we have certain conditions for either wanting that or not? What might we expect?

We might anticipate many of the problems we would face then because we already have them: crowding, disease, and poverty; shortages of food, energy, and other resources; and acceleration of environmental contamination and global warming. Problems related to productivity, economic contributions to society, and leisure will be exaggerated over what they are currently. If I will live to 200, should I work until I am 175? Or, if I retire earlier, say, at 65 as I might now, what will I do with the next 135 years? If we have not licked the disease and disability problems associated with aging, how many of us will wholly or partially depend on others and for how long? And the others who care for us, will they be taken from the "productive" portion of society, as measured by something like the Gross National Product, but still will be essential to the overall success of most of us living 200 years?

New issues could arise related to multigenerational families. Now, the distinctions among the three or four generations that exist in many families—young children, parents, grandparents, perhaps great-grandparents—seem relatively clear. The mindsets, world views, concerns, attitudes, and behaviors of children, parents, and grandparents, although they have some commonalities, are discernable and often can be assigned to one generation or another. In a family of eight or ten generations, however, assuming the process of maturing to adulthood takes no longer than it does now, and the process of dying is about the same, more people will populate the "middle" generations and the differences among the generations will be small.

Some people think it is unnatural or not God's will to tinker with the natural processes of dying and death. If nature or God intended us to live 200 years, then we would be living that long now. (My apologies, but this book is not the place to debate people's various beliefs.) But humankind has tried to subvert the natural order, with variable success, since prehistory. Do not setting broken bones, immunizing with vaccines, prescribing antibiotics, removing inflamed appendices, opening clogged arteries, implanting fertilized eggs into a woman who otherwise could not have a child, administering potent medications for a failing heart, connecting a patient who would likely die of respiratory failure to a ventilator, all constitute an intervention in the natural order? Where do we separate what is acceptable from what is not? Should we draw the line at adjusting the genetic code?

Whether or not you personally draw the line at manipulating the genetic code, science already crossed that line a long time ago. We are well into the era of expanding our understanding of genetic information, seeking to manipulate it, and acting on it to create a desirable baby, reverse or ameliorate genetic disorders, treat certain cancers, or, as we talked about before, control the aging process and prolong life. Also, so-called precision medicine, sometimes called personalized medicine, relies on knowing an individual's unique genetic makeup to guide prevention and treatment that is tailored specifically to that person.

This is a lot to assimilate and make up our minds about. It turns out, according to a poll of US adults, that people have mixed views on emerging genetic techniques and what they are intended to achieve.[11] Most people approve of using genetic technology to prevent and treat serious diseases, but few think it is right to improve intelligence or create desirable physical traits, so-called designer babies, through editing of the reproductive genes. Regarding the prospect of living beyond 120 years, another poll indicated that 56% of Americans would not want treatments that would allow them to live to 120 years, whereas 38% would want them (6% were noncommittal).[12] Nearly 70% felt that the ideal length of life was 79 to 100 years.

When I ask people informally whether they would want to live 200 years, the responses almost always hinge on concerns about quality of life. If a person has had or anticipates having a significant diminution in their quality of life, however they define that for themselves (see Chapter 2), they may see more years as an additional burden to be avoided. If a person sees a longer life, accompanied largely by having solved the problems of aging and of society, and sustaining a good quality of life, then additional years may seem more attractive. Socioeconomic status plays into this assessment as well—if you have trouble making ends meet during your first 100 years, you cannot look forward to as comfortable a second 100 years as someone who always had what she needed. Likewise, people with families or communities surrounding them who would care for and support them might have a brighter view of the future, regardless of whether it's for the period of old age that we now have or an extended one in the future.

So, do I want to live 200 years? Well, it depends, doesn't it? If I can live most of that time in good health and keep my wits, and if the world is a decent place in which to live, that could be very nice. But if my body deteriorates and my mind doesn't work, and I must live in a hostile environment, I don't want it.

DYING AT HOME IS SO OLD FASHIONED

In the introduction I described my earliest memory, of standing with my father when I was three years old during my grandmother's wake, which took place in the front room of her home. She had died quickly after a stroke in her mid-seventies. She was in the company of her husband, her children and grandchildren, and other relatives and friends. She was not hospitalized and the gadgetry that is associated now with end-of-life events did not exist. Her dying and death seem uncomplicated and straightforward compared to the dying process for many people now.

In contrast, consider this contemporary experience with the dying process. Shirley, a 72-year-old woman has lived with the diagnosis of recurrent breast cancer for several years. At first, she responded to treatment, but four months ago she developed back and chest pain and metastases to the spine and ribs were discovered. Since then she has dwindled, losing appetite and mobility. Three weeks ago, she began to cough and have difficulty breathing and was admitted to the hospital with pneumonia. A chest X-ray showed probable metastases to the lung. Now, in the intensive care unit (ICU), she receives potent antibiotics and she cannot think clearly enough to make medical decisions for herself. Shirley's husband of 45 years attends her constantly. A son and daughter visit frequently.

The medical team explains the poor outlook to the family and seeks direction. Should DNR and DNI orders be written? What about surgically placing a feeding tube into her stomach to provide nutrition? The family is undecided at first but, because Shirley cannot swallow food or fluids, they allow the doctors to insert a feeding tube. Later, as Shirley's breathing becomes more distressed and her blood oxygen plummets, the family agrees to having an endotracheal tube passed through her mouth into the trachea and connected to a mechanical ventilator.

Two more weeks pass, and the medical team again raises questions. Where are we going with this? What are the goals of treatment? Should we continue with the treatments and add new ones as medical indications change? If we continue mechanical ventilation, because of the damaging effects of the endotracheal tube on the trachea over a week or so, the endotracheal tube will need to be replaced by a surgical tracheostomy, a hole through the front of the neck directly into the trachea to which the ventilator is attached. What were Shirley's wishes about such things before she became ill? Her husband, with much reluctance, accepts that it is time to let go. The daughter agrees, saying, "Mom would not want to live like this." But the son says, "No! Mom always was a fighter. She would want to beat this." Shirley, like over half of Americans, did not appoint a health care proxy agent to represent her wishes if she could not speak for herself, or make her wishes known in some other explicit way by writing a living will or by discussing end-of-life matters with her loved ones. The family is left to resolve their disagreements, during a time of emotional distress and pressure to "do something," as best they can. We will talk about making our wishes known, including appointing a health care proxy agent and creating a living will, in Chapter 3.

My grandmother's life seems to have approached an ideal, rarely achieved but sometimes approximated, in which one lives a long, healthy life and then drops dead. She was fortunate to have lived to her seventies. Many of her birth contemporaries had died of illness and other causes that perhaps could have been prevented by public health improvements and recent medical treatments, had they been available. Shirley, however, regardless of how healthy she might have been before she developed breast cancer, entered a phase that my grandmother could not have experienced. Shirley of course benefited from what contemporary medicine could offer her. But at the same time, she progressively experienced several circumstances that characterize present-day end of life. As she approached the end of her life, her health and quality of life began to deteriorate slowly, then rapidly and inexorably. She became the recipient of the marvels of contemporary medicine, which provide plenty of options to hold her death at bay and keep the spark of life aglow, and she entered an ambiguous and scary territory for which she and her loved ones had not prepared.

Several generations ago most people died at home. This is because that is where people had died for centuries and being in a hospital as one was dying offered little additional benefit. Very little could be done in the hospital that could not be done at home. And hospitals sometimes were dangerous places where patients acquired new infections for which there was no specific treatment. (Hospital-acquired infections continue to be a problem now, which is one reason to try to make one's stay in the hospital as brief as possible.) However, as diagnostics and treatments advanced, if one were to participate in them, one had to be in a hospital.

Although 80% of Americans say they would prefer to die at home, about 60% die in hospitals and about 20% die in nursing homes; only about 20% die at home.[1] It is easy to see why this might occur. I would like to die at home, but when I become sick with a lethal disease or when a complication of that disease develops, the usual place for much of the treatment is in a hospital. One thing leads to another and it may be impractical or impossible to discharge me to home. The advent of hospice and palliative care (Chapter 5) have allowed more dying patients to go home or at least receive more personal, tender care in the presence of loved ones. Further, we can express our wishes about end-of-life care through our health care proxy agent, a living will, or a POLST document (Physician's Orders for Life-Sustaining Treatment, sometimes called MOLST, Medical Order for Life-Sustaining Treatment), which we will discuss in Chapter 3 when we talk about making our wishes about end-of-life matters known in advance. Whether you die at home, in a hospital, or in a nursing home, it seems that the important common elements should be respect for your wishes, attention to your physical and emotional comfort, and respect for your dignity, along with opportunities for friends and loved ones to be present.

Our technology, which usually is credited with saving lives and restoring health, also has created new types of suffering, for the patient, for family and friends, and sometimes for the health professionals who care for them. The patient may or may not suffer in the conventional sense of experiencing pain and discomfort, but even when a person is unconscious, there can be a loss of dignity and suffering in an existential way. Loved ones feel this and may be distressed. And I have sat in conferences in which health care professionals—nurses, doctors, respiratory therapists, and others—express their frustration, anxiety, and sadness when decision-makers for such patients want to continue what the health professionals consider to be futile treatments that seem to prolong the suffering and indignity of the patient. We will examine this problem more when we talk about quality of life and making our wishes known in Chapters 2 and 3.

For myself, even if I am not dying, like the large majority of readers of this book, I expect, I prefer to be at home rather than in the hospital. Home usually is a more comfortable and comforting place to be. In addition, however, as a physician with over four decades experience with hospitals, sometimes as a patient myself, I know that even in the modern era, hospital-acquired infections and other mishaps befall hospitalized patients. I want to be in the hospital if I have to be, but I want to be home as quickly as it is medically safe. And I have made it clear to my loved ones, if at all possible, that I would like to die at home.

DYING IS EXPENSIVE

Spending on health care is concentrated at the end of life. Whereas dying at home used to be attended with little fuss and expense, now end-of-life care accounts for about 10% of all health care spending and evokes the gadgetry of current diagnostics and therapies, which carry a high price tag and usually occur in a hospital.

In 2011, 7% of the civilian population of the United States who were not living in institutions were hospitalized at one time or another. As one would expect, older people comprise a higher proportion of hospitalized patients. Also, according to a 2015 report from the Kaiser Family Foundation, of the 2.5 million people who die each year, as expected, three-quarters of them are over age 65.[2] This means that Medicare is the largest insurer of health care during the last year of life. Medicare expenses during that last year of life account for about one-quarter of total Medicare spending for health care. Of course, many elderly people have multiple serious and complex conditions, which adds to the high cost of health care in the last year of life.[2-4]

Hospitalization is an expensive form of health care. Hospital charges, which vary in different regions of the country and from hospital to hospital, are not the same as what the insurance company or Medicare pays. Insurance payments are negotiated rates, generally are lower than the charges, and may not cover the actual costs to the hospital for providing the billed services. Patients without insurance usually are billed the full charges. If you are very wealthy and do not have health insurance, paying the hospital bill may not be a problem for you. However, most affluent people have health insurance. The large majority of people without health insurance are of modest means or are poor, and a small portion are legally undocumented workers. Often people without insurance can make arrangements with the hospital to pay the bill, sometimes adjusted, over time. Also, patients without insurance who are eligible for Medicaid, a program that currently is shared between the Federal Government and each state to provide some health care coverage for people with low incomes, typically receive advice from the hospital to enroll in Medicaid.

Regardless of how the hospital bill is paid, hospital charges associated with an ordinary hospitalization are substantial and being in an ICU adds more expense. A study of over 250 hospitals across the United States showed that the average length of stay in an ICU was about nine days for patients not requiring respiratory ventilation. Treatment with ventilation, which occurred in about one-third of the ICU patients, added significantly to the length of stay, averaging about 15 days.[13] Some hospitals post their charges for various services. For example, University Hospitals of Cleveland lists a charge for "room and board" of $6,285 per day in their medical or surgical ICU.[14] An average stay of 15 days would amount to over $94,000. In a typical hospital, the patient can expect to receive additional bills from physicians for professional services.

The costs of hospitalization are sobering for individuals, and even though we may not pay the bill directly, we pay it through insurance premiums, Medicare withholdings, and taxes that help support public programs such as Medicaid and health care for veterans. Current total health care spending in the United States is about $3.5 trillion per year and, in the aggregate, costs of hospitalization account for about 30% of that. Incidentally, the $3.5 trillion we spend annually for health care in this country is over 17% of the country's Gross Domestic Product

(GDP). This is much higher in both absolute amount and percent of GDP than any other country. Earlier we talked about how poorly the United States compares with other industrialized countries in some measures of health, such as life expectancy. Are we getting our money's worth?

The substantial contribution of the dying process to the costs of health care in the United States raises questions not only about whether such expenditures can be reduced, but also whether the savings could be applied elsewhere, say, to providing other benefits to people covered by Medicare who are not dying or perhaps to people somewhere else along the trajectory of life, such as children who need vaccines and other medical services. Where would you spend the money that was saved by reducing end-of-life expenses? Perhaps somewhere else in health care or for another purpose entirely?

The data relating to expenditures in the last year of life, of course, are derived retrospectively, after people have died. Prospectively, months in advance of death, we do not know for sure just when someone will die. Some people benefit from the expensive treatments and return home or elsewhere to continue living. Some of those even recover a sufficient quality of life to make the time, effort, and expense seem justified. The end of life comes later.

But we do know, with little uncertainty, that when someone is very sick, is on a ventilator, for example, and receiving other expensive treatments, and the situation is futile, that death is imminent. Here the situation becomes one of acting according to the person's values and an understanding of the realistic predicted medical outcome—concerns that are shared among the dying person, loved ones, and the medical care team.

Some individuals and families of patients want "everything done." People who take this stance sometimes do not understand what "everything" actually means and what are the capabilities and limitations of "everything." Or they may understand what "everything" means but still want all life sustaining measures because they believe that the spark of life is more important than perceptions of quality of life.

Others feel that there are limits to what even modern medicine and science can do to restore an acceptable quality of life or halt an irreversible process that is leading to death. They acknowledge that death comes to everyone and now may be the time to accept that eventuality.

How would you confront these difficult questions? How can you, particularly if you enjoy good health now, assess what will matter to you at the end of life? What does quality of life mean to you, and how does it figure into making your wishes known about matters at the end of life? We will explore these questions in the chapters ahead.

Chapter 2

THE GOOD LIFE . . . AND WHAT DOES THE QUALITY OF MY LIFE MEAN TO ME?

From time to time I declare that I want to live a rectangular life. It is true that I am tall and somewhat angular, but I am not relating a rectangular life to my appearance nor to any behavior or way of thinking. I refer to how my life might appear on a graph that relates years lived on the horizontal axis to some index of quality of life on the vertical axis (Figure 2.1). I want to live a long life, but a life in which I remain well and mentally active for as long as possible. Then, I want to die quickly, without lingering or suffering or creating a burden for my family. Thus, in a two-dimensional graphic depiction of my life, I would begin high on the vertical axis at birth and remain as high as possible until, after many years, I would die suddenly and the line would plunge to zero, resembling a rectangle. Of course, a quick death at an early age, or beginning life in poor health partway up the

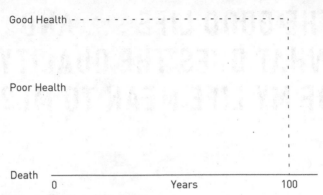

Good Health ─ ─ ─ ─ ─ ─ ─ ─ ─ ─ ─ ─ ─ ─ ┐

Poor Health

Death ────────────────────────────
     0   Years   100

Figure 2.1. The Rectangular Life.

vertical scale but dying over a short time later in life, could result in a rectangular life, but I don't want those options. I want it all—a long life that begins healthy and stays that way, and is exciting and full of mental and physical vigor, and then, done.

Everyone knows that this is not how life turns out for anyone. Even the healthiest people who die at an advanced age have some functional diminution—things don't work as well as they did at 25—so the horizontal line tapers inexorably down. For many, the downward trajectory is more pronounced. And, thanks to the so-called miracles of contemporary medicine, for some of us the life line trails lower and lower and lower for a long time. The rectangular life is an ideal.

So what is quality of life? Aristotle declared that "The quality of life is determined by its activities." And according to

Martin Luther King Jr., "The quality, not the longevity, of one's life is what is important."

If you ask a health professional about quality of life, you might get something related to the HRQOL, Health Related Quality of Life, which is a quantitative and statistical assessment of a person's well-being, taking into account bodily, emotional, cognitive, social, and sometimes spiritual aspects of a person's life, and how well-being may be affected by disease and disability. The HRQOL is used not only to assess an individual's quality of life but also the quality of life of groups of people, such as the residents of a country or a demographic group.

Most of us, however, receive the question about quality of life in a personal way. What gives my life meaning? What do I enjoy doing? How satisfied am I with my life? Would the diminution in my satisfaction in life or the relinquishing of anything I am capable of doing now influence decisions I may have to make at the end of life? Each of us views our life and the quality of it in ways that are unique to us.

Ask any number of people what they mean by quality of life and you will hear as many definitions. People's thoughts about quality of life vary greatly and depend on what they value in their day-to-day lives. As I have interacted over the years with people from a wide range of vocations, ages, and backgrounds, I've heard views such as these.

"If by quality of my life you mean, what do I enjoy doing, well, there are lots of things. I play basketball a lot, go camping when

I can with my family. I have a great wife and three kids, a boy 12, a girl 10, a girl 6. And I like my work, and am proud of it."

"I grew up on my farm. I know that I am unusual. Everyone in my high school class has either left this area or gone into something other than farming. I love it. I can't imagine doing anything else."

"I still enjoy the thrill of greeting new students each fall. Teaching is very challenging, but it helps define who I am. As a teacher I am doing something important and useful. It certainly is a big part of the quality of my life."

"I get a great deal of satisfaction and enjoyment from my grandchildren. I have two sets, two kids about an hour away and another two about four hours away. I think the things that affected my quality of life have changed gradually over the years, but right now it seems that being with my grandchildren and continuing some of the relationships I have had for years and traveling are important."

I also have found that people who are commonly considered by the non-disabled to be disabled describe their quality of life in much the same way as I would as a non-disabled person. For example, patients have said things to me such as:

"I don't think of myself as being disabled. I am able in a different way. Because I am blind, I see things differently. Maybe that is an advantage to me. The quality of my life is very good. I enjoy my job as a social worker, I enjoy my friends, I enjoy listening to birds and being outdoors, I enjoy reading."

"I was shocked and depressed after the accident that paralyzed me below the chest. I had never thought about something like this happening to me. For a while I didn't want to go on. But I got better and had a lot of support from my family and boyfriend. Now I've got a good job, a husband and little boy, and, you know, it could be a lot worse. Yes, I would say the quality of my life is pretty good."

The performance of both physical and mental functions seems integral to our concepts of quality of life. When I ask people how they would define quality of life for themselves, predictably, each person's notion of quality of life involves some mix of physical and intellectual function. Many say something like, "I think being able to think and speak are the most important. I dread becoming demented." When I ask how they would feel about being paralyzed and bedridden but still able to think normally, that provokes some re-examination of the primacy of cognitive function. My wife said once, "If I ever get that way, terminate me." To her, "that way" involves some horrifying compromise of cognitive function—such as being demented or in a medical condition with no ability to think or recognize people. By the way, terminating her might solve her problem, but would create new ones for me.

Whether we think we would not want to live "that way" depends largely on the specifics of our anticipated disability. Further, notions of quality of life are influenced by perceived or experienced symptoms of illness, side effects of treatment, and limitations in physical or mental activities (e.g., walking, eating, reading, interacting with relatives and friends, listening to music, watching television). Also, a person's regard for dignity and independence are highly relevant.

Our ideas about quality of life usually are based largely on the state of physical and mental health to which we have become accustomed. Conditions that we perceive as severely compromising our quality of life are related to an anticipated change in our current condition. If we are able in mind and body now, what we think might severely compromise our quality of life and be intolerable may not be so if we actually become disabled in some way. Humans are remarkably resilient. It is common for people with chronic illness or significant disability to view their quality of life as being better than what others think about their quality of life. People often learn to cope with diminished abilities and compensate for them. We may get a glimpse of that in the adjustments that most of us make as we accommodate to the diminishments of aging. For many, aging is similar in kind, but different in degree, to acquiring disabilities. In a sense everyone becomes disabled to some degree, and if we view ourselves as not disabled, that is a temporary condition.

For some people, sustaining biological life is of paramount importance and so-called quality of life is of little consequence. They hold that life must be preserved even if the person's medical condition cannot be meaningfully improved. This view may come from personal conviction or religious belief. Sometimes it is because the person or the loved ones of that person are hopeful of improvement or recovery, even when the outlook seems futile.

It is risky to confer our own views about quality of life on others. For example, some parents who know that their unborn child has trisomy 21 (Down syndrome) anticipate a lower than acceptable quality of life for the child and a burden on the family if the child is born, and they choose abortion. Other parents choose to raise children and adults with Down syndrome and do all they can to help provide their children with a good quality of life. They are eager to raise such a child in a caring environment.

The physician Anna Reisman tells a wonderful story of the perceived quality of life of a severely physically and mentally disabled woman, her own sister Deborah, and the gift of her life to others.[1] Deborah was born with tuberous sclerosis, a rare genetic disorder that causes benign tumors in the brain and other organs and, in Deborah's case, seizures, severe mental disability, and inability to speak. Deborah died at age 40 and had lived the last 25 years of her life in a group home, "spending most of her time sitting on a favorite brown leather chair, legs tucked under her, eyes focused on nothing in particular."

> "Deborah was elegant in her own way, slim with thick, shiny, dark hair. In her skinny jeans and Aeropostale sweatshirts, she looked like a pretty teenager even in her 40s. Sometimes she was willing to interact with family, housemates, and caregivers—clapping her hands excitedly in imitation of me or one of my kids, tolerating a game of catch (from her

armchair, with a half-deflated yellow basketball), or standing and grasping my forearm en route to the snack cabinet."

After Deborah's death, Dr. Reisman and another sister, Lisa, arranged a memorial service for Deborah. They worried whether anyone other than closest family would attend and whether anyone would say something in remembrance of Deborah.

"As it turned out, about 30 showed up, and plenty spoke. There was one caregiver who read a lovely acrostic poem she'd written about Deborah, and others who recalled sweet and funny moments from her last few years. There were people who'd worked at Deborah's group home many years earlier who still thought about her. There was the sister of one of her housemates who said that her sister and Deborah had been best friends. (I'd never realized that Deborah was capable of having a friend.) Her primary care doctor, who had visited her in emergency departments, hospitals, and her home, spoke movingly about how much she had learned in the challenging process of caring for her.

"So many people referred to her as a gift. I started to understand that they were talking about selfless love, about how she made people feel good without doing much of anything, simply by being there, sitting on her chair and offering an occasional smile or joyful laugh."

So, perceptions of quality of life, whether they occur in anticipation of a new life, in reflection of one's own life or the life of another, or in contemplation of the end of life, are complex and distinctive for each of us. Those perceptions affect how we plan for the end of life and make end-of-life decisions, which we will take up in the next chapter.

Chapter 3
MAKING OUR WISHES KNOWN

And when Jacob had made an end of commanding his sons, he
gathered up his feet into the bed, and yielded up the ghost, and
was gathered unto his people.

—Genesis 49:33, the Bible

I don't know whether Jacob's life was rectangular in the sense we
talked about in Chapter 2, but this passage from Genesis describes
the ideal that many of us would want for ourselves—as death
approaches we make our wishes known to those who matter to us,
we hop into bed, and die. If being gathered unto our people means
going to heaven, then that, too. This approximates a mode of death that
was experienced as recently as two generations ago but does not describe the manner in which most people die in contemporary America.
We talked about this at length in Chapter 1. We cannot return to a
former time, of course, but we can do things to ensure that our last days
and weeks and months are as close as possible to the way we would
want them. We can make our wishes known in advance.

Most of us want to make decisions about our lives for ourselves throughout our lives. Dying, that important part of life before we die, often is protracted and complicated. Decisions usually are required during that time, and we want to have some control over the decisions that need to be made then. Some of the big ones might be: Do I want this treatment or that? Should I be resuscitated if my heart stops? Do I want to have a tube in my trachea? Would I choose to have intravenous (IV) fluids and a feeding tube? (Some people, for religious or other reasons, agree to stop all treatments under certain conditions, except they draw the line at IV fluids and nutrition—they want those continued.) Do I want to remain in the hospital or go home? Or do I not want to be treated in the hospital at all?

But what if we are unable to make those decisions ourselves? What if our condition prevents us from being able to decide, because of either the illness itself or our cognitive decline for other reasons? Then how do these decisions get made? Who makes them?

We can plan for this and give our loved ones and physicians and others some idea of what we might want by what are called advance directives. Preferably, we would document our advance directives by designating a health care proxy (HCP) agent or creating a living will. Lacking a written document, advance directives may be interpreted from conversations or explicit oral statements that we have made to family and friends about our end-of-life wishes so that people who need to decide about our care have some guidance about what we would want.

AUTONOMY—THE RIGHT TO DECIDE FOR MYSELF

Before we look at ways in which you might make your wishes known in advance, let's take a few moments to explore the concept of autonomy. It is an important idea because it pertains not only to making decisions at the end of life but to nearly all aspects of life.

We cherish our autonomy. Autonomy is the right to make decisions for ourselves—something that humans have valued in various contexts throughout history. The application of autonomy to the patient–physician relationship is relatively new, however, as it did not seem important at all over centuries of medical practice.

Hippocrates, who lived about 2,500 years ago, gave us many of the principles that guide physicians and health care professionals today, such as, act in the best interest of the patient, seek to do good (beneficence), avoid harm (non-maleficence), and don't talk about patients outside of the patient–physician relationship (confidentiality). But Hippocrates would be unfamiliar with our contemporary notion that patients should make, or even be capable of making, decisions for themselves. The presumption that the physician, who is the repository of all relevant medical knowledge and judgment, knows best—so-called paternalism—prevailed until recently and persists sometimes today. Paternalism presumes that the patient does not have the capacity to understand complex medical issues sufficiently to make decisions about them, or at least the patient's place is not to do that.

This has changed. We now believe that most people do have the capacity to make medical decisions, when properly informed, and we regard doing so to be a person's right. This is consistent with the notion of having the right to make our own decisions in all aspects of our lives. We believe that rights are crucial to people living freely and being respected by the state and other citizens. In America especially, rights are clung to fiercely, and we cite the centuries-old Bill of Rights in everything from friendly discussions of current events to political elections. It would be no exaggeration to say that the notion of having rights is in the cultural DNA of the United States, as it is in many parts of the world.

We also live in an era of access to vast amounts of information, some inaccurate, but much actually quite reliable, particularly when retrieved from respected websites. Such knowledge, plus a higher level of education on average, enables patients to participate better in decision-making for their medical care. Physicians need to respect the input of patients as they work with them in developing a plan of management of their medical condition.

Here are two clinical situations that show how autonomy might play out in an awkward or problematic way in the relationship between a patient and a physician.

1. Darren, a 68-year-old man with a several-year history of increasing difficulty urinating, consults Dr. Bradley, a urologist. Dr. Bradley performs a rectal examination and detects a large prostate, which would be expected in a man Darren's age, and a small nodule on the prostate. However, a biopsy of the prostate shows a low-grade prostate cancer, which typically is slowly progressive.

Some experts advise against treatment of some low-grade prostate cancers because, depending on the person's age and other medical conditions, statistically the person may die of something else before he dies of prostate cancer and treatment of the prostate cancer may be associated with serious side effects. Dr. Bradley, in discussing further management of the cancer with Darren, offers several options, including so-called watchful waiting, radiation, and surgery. He explains the benefits and risks of each option and says, "It's up to you, Darren. Which one do you want?"

What is the proper balance of the autonomy of the patient with the responsibility of the physician to offer expert professional advice? To what extent should the decision-making process be shared between the patient and physician? This question is widely discussed in medical education and among physicians. In my view, shared decision-making integrates both a respect for the autonomy of the patient and acknowledgment of the expertise of the physician. When I consult my doctor, yes, I want to decide for myself, after I understand my condition and know the risks and benefits of various treatments. But I also expect my physician to give me her informed opinion. She is the expert. That is why I went to see her. If my physician thinks a particular treatment is best for me, I want her to tell me and explain why. Then I can decide. If two or more treatments seem about equal, I want to know why that is the case.

2. Lila, an 83-year-old woman, has had rectal bleeding for three weeks. Her daughter brings her to Dr. Lindsay, a gastroenterologist. The daughter tells Dr. Lindsay in private that if the diagnosis is cancer,

"Please don't tell my mother." Colonoscopy reveals a lower colon growth. Biopsies confirm a colon cancer. CT scan shows enlarged abdominal lymph nodes and several spots in the liver. All this suggests advanced colon cancer with spread to the lymph nodes and the liver. Dr. Lindsay schedules a meeting with Lila and her daughter to discuss further management.

This story raises important questions regarding the autonomy of the patient, of course, but also truth telling and family culture. Should Dr. Lindsay comply with the daughter's request and not tell Lila her diagnosis and prognosis? Does Lila have the right to know her diagnosis? Most of us would say she does. But is her family or culture one that accepts a certain amount of shielding of older or vulnerable people against bad news? My approach to this would be to have responded at the beginning to the daughter's request to withhold bad news from her mother by saying something like, "In my practice I believe that each patient has the right to know his or her diagnosis and prognosis. Let's talk about how this applies to your mother." This will initiate a discussion about how we would share important information with the patient. Only in rare circumstances, such as the high likelihood of harm to the patient if she knew the diagnosis, would I withhold essential information from her.

These accounts suggest that, although our culture places a high value on knowing about our own health and making decisions for ourselves, each person's situation is unique, and sometimes autonomy has to be defined for our special circumstances. Further, to be autonomous in our decision-making includes having the right, and perhaps the obligation, to think through some of the possibilities we may face at the end of life and to declare in advance how we would like those possibilities to be handled.

DECISION-MAKING CAPACITY

In order to express our autonomy and make decisions for ourselves, we must have the mental capacity to do so. Earlier I said that we believe that most people have the capacity to make decisions, when properly informed. But not all people. Some, because of illness, a psychiatric condition, insufficient mental development, dementia, or other cognitive disorder, are not able to make decisions. Also, some people can make some decisions, but not other decisions, and their decision-making capacity may fluctuate.

Decision-making capacity depends on one's ability to understand a situation and the consequences of the decision. In a medical context, one needs to know the reasons, the intended outcome, and the benefits and the risks of any intervention. Some of us can make small decisions but not more consequential ones. We all make many decisions throughout every day, most of them trivial, some more important. After I awakened this morning, I decided what clothes to wear and what to have for breakfast. I usually have Cheerios, so that is not much of a decision for me. I may have decided for myself, or decided to allow someone else to decide on my behalf, what I will do at various times today. If I have a bad cold or respiratory infection, I may decide to see my primary care physician, or put it off in the hope I will feel better tomorrow. If I see her, she may recommend certain things to do for my complaints, about which I need to decide. Someday I may be required to make more complicated and consequential decisions, such as those that involve medical and surgical treatments for more serious and perhaps life-threatening conditions.

Another term, competence, also is used to characterize a person's ability to decide and sometimes is used interchangeably with decision-making capacity. Someone might say, "She is not competent to make that decision." I generally do not use competence in a health care setting but reserve it for legal judgments about a person's mental capacities. Generally, mental competence is something that a magistrate rules on and may extend beyond medical situations to include the ability to manage financial matters and other aspects of a person's life.

In a health care situation, how do we determine whether a person has decision-making capacity for the decision at hand? In some situations, it is easy. A person in a coma, or who suffers from delirium, or who has severe developmental cognitive disability, or advanced dementia, or the like, clearly cannot make any decisions. However, in the case of someone with mild dementia or poor ability to grasp facts and consequences, but who still has been able to take some responsibility for himself, it is not always immediately evident that that person can or cannot make a particular decision.

The responsibility to make the determination of decision-making capacity falls to the attending physician, the physician who is mainly in charge of the patient's care, whether it is in the hospital or elsewhere. The attending physician judges whether the person can understand the particular situation for which a decision is required, the intended outcome, and the likely benefits and risks. The attending physician may seek advice from other physicians or health care professionals. Sometimes psychiatrists and ethics consultants are asked to advise on a patient's ability to make decisions because those professionals generally have experience in dealing with people who have impairments in decision-making capacity. But it is the attending physician's job to determine decision-making capacity, with or without the advice of others.

Consider this example of how a person's decision-making capacity is not always obvious and needs to be determined in the context of the specific decision at hand. Maria, a 66-year-old woman, had lived for several years in a nursing home because she could not take care of herself, largely due to early onset dementia. She became confused from time to time, had difficulty remembering recent events, and could not manage her own financial affairs. She also had several medical problems, including poorly controlled diabetes, high blood pressure, and serious heart disease. However, she was able to dress and feed herself, walk, and otherwise care for herself. One day on the way back to her room from lunch Maria fell in the hallway and struck her back. When she was brought to the emergency department, X-rays showed that she had fractured several vertebrae. She was admitted to the hospital, where the orthopedic surgeons recommended spine surgery, although they acknowledged that the risks of surgery were high because of the patient's diabetes and heart disease.

Did Maria have the capacity to make the decision at hand, whether to have surgery or not? Could she grasp the facts of her situation, did she understand what the surgery was intended to do, and was she able to balance the risks of the surgery against the intended benefits? It seemed unlikely that she could do any of those things as well as if she had not been demented, yet she knew what she wanted and what she did not want when the recommendation of surgery was put to her. She was clear that she did not want surgery. She wanted to return to the nursing home, which she regarded as her home. She was willing to tolerate her back pain, and she said she would take her chances without surgery. She had no HCP agent or relative who could be called upon to act as a decision-maker for her.

The attending physician, with the input from an ethics consultant, determined that Maria had sufficient mental capacity to make this decision and discharged her to her nursing home on appropriate pain medications. The attending physician took into account Maria's expressed wishes despite the limitation in her decision-making capacity, the higher risks of surgery, and the practicality of performing a complicated operation against the patient's will, one that would be followed by weeks of immobilization and rehabilitation.

What would have been the attending physician's determination if some of the facts of this case were different? What if the patient did have an HCP or other surrogate decision-maker? What would that person have said on her behalf? What if the patient were a better surgical risk? What if the patient had had another condition for which the treatment was something else, such as long-term kidney dialysis or an in-hospital course of intravenous antibiotic therapy, each with different risks and degrees of cooperation required by the patient? The variables of the specific decision at hand need to be taken into account by the family, surrogate decision-makers if they exist, and the physicians.

Another patient had trouble expressing herself, which raised the question of whether she had lost decision-making capacity because of it. Sarah was a 54-year-old woman who had suffered a stroke due to a ruptured blood vessel aneurysm in her brain. For several weeks afterward, she was unable to speak or write, but she did seem able to respond "yes" or "no" to simple questions by blinking her eyes. Her son, who was her HCP agent and had been close to his mother, seemed to know her wishes and understand her responses. Ordinarily, if the attending physician had determined that Sarah had decisional capacity, her son as HCP agent would not have made decisions for her. On the other hand, if she had been determined to have lost decisional capacity, her son would be empowered to make decisions for her. In this case, the attending physician felt that Sarah did have decisional capacity, but it was difficult communicating with her. So, although technically the son could not function in the capacity of HCP agent, for practical purposes the attending physician regarded Sarah and her son together as the decision-maker.

The end of life includes many decision points. Do I want this or that treatment, given the circumstances of my condition? Do I want palliative care? Should I go to the hospital or stay home? But what if I lose my ability to make decisions? Who will make those decisions for me? And will they make the decisions as I might have if I still had the capacity to make them? That is where advance directives come in.

ADVANCE DIRECTIVES

Now that we have established some concepts that are relevant to end-of-life decisions—the right to make our own decisions and the mental capacity to do so, or lack thereof—let's talk about ways in which we can make our wishes known through advance directives. In the United States, less than 30% of the population has completed advance directives.[1] If you don't already have an advance directive, perhaps after reading this you will feel encouraged to create one soon! It is probably easier than you think.

Health Care Proxy Agents

One way we can anticipate the need to make critical decisions at the end of our lives and make sure that there is a plan in place even if we are not able to make health decisions for ourselves, is by naming an HCP agent ahead of time. In some states this is called a medical or health care power of attorney or a durable power of attorney for health care. Sometimes the term "health care proxy" is used to mean the person who is the HCP agent. Sometimes "health care proxy" means the document or form that names the HCP agent and may include other stipulations. When a person loses the capacity to make health care decisions, an HCP agent tries to preserve that person's autonomy by making decisions as close as possible to what the person would have made.

Being an HCP agent is a big responsibility. If you are someone's HCP agent, you are empowered to make medical decisions for that person under certain conditions. One important condition is that the person, who once had the capacity to make medical decisions, has lost that capacity. However, the HCP agent does not have the authority to determine whether the person has lost decision-making capacity, meaning, the HCP agent cannot say when he or she would begin to function as the HCP agent. That authority rests with the physician in charge of the patient, as I said earlier when we talked about autonomy.

After a physician determines that a person no longer has decision-making capacity, then the HCP agent can begin to make health care decisions for that person. So, the designated HCP agent should not make decisions for the person if the person still can make decisions.

For example, if your husband is your HCP agent and you still have the capacity to make decisions, he, of course, as your husband could help you make decisions, or not, as you wish. You would still make your own medical decisions. Once you lose decisional capacity, your husband, as your HCP agent, is authorized to make medical decisions for you. However, unless you specifically name your husband or wife as your HCP agent, he or she will not automatically be your HCP agent. It is likely, however, that, according to the laws of most states, one's spouse would be eligible to be the surrogate decision-maker. Later, I discuss the reasons why you might want to designate a specific HCP agent for yourself rather than simply letting the law decide for you who will make your health care decisions.

Another condition that your HCP agent must respect is that he or she is obligated to make decisions for you according to your wishes, not their own wishes. It is almost as if your HCP agent becomes you for the purposes of making your decisions. This sometimes is a difficult concept for HCP agents to understand. They may want to decide on the basis of their own values and interests. But they should not do that. They should decide according to what you would want. Of course, it is convenient if the HCP agent and the person for whom the HCP agent is speaking have similar values and interests.

This requirement, to act according to the wishes of the person who has lost decisional capacity, presupposes that the HCP agent knows the wishes of that person. Thus, if you are selecting an HCP agent, you will want to have conversations with that person to make sure he or she understands your wishes. Or, conversely, if someone asks you to be their HCP agent, you will want to talk with them to understand their values and wishes about end-of-life situations. Because the exact medical situation that the person will experience and the HCP agent will face is difficult to predict, these conversations provide a broad mutual understanding of the kinds of things that might happen and give the HCP agent guidance.

Sometimes HCP agents do not know the wishes of the person who has lost decisional capacity, usually because they did not fully understand the obligations of being an HCP agent. When the person and HCP agent have not had explicit discussions on these matters, the HCP agent should make decisions based on what the HCP agent understands are the person's values and beliefs from previous association with that person. Sometimes the HCP agent comes to know the person's wishes by talking with others. Thus, anyone with information about the person's wishes, such as a relative, a friend, a physician or nurse, should be encouraged to share it with the HCP agent and the clinicians taking care of the patient if the HCP agent has not had those discussions with the patient. Only when the HCP agent cannot determine the patient's wishes or values, either because there have been no previous conversations with the patient, or there is no previously executed document, or other relatives and friends cannot provide enlightenment, should the HCP agent decide according to what the HCP agent believes are in the patient's best interests.

The distinction between so-called best interests of a person and the wishes of that person is sometimes important. Often they are the same. For example, in the course of ordinary medical care, a physician recommends antibiotics, in what the physician believes are the best interests of the patient, and the patient agrees. Or a physician recommends open heart surgery and the patient agrees. A physician recommends kidney dialysis, or a feeding tube, or a tracheostomy (a tube in the trachea for breathing), and the patient agrees. But sometimes a person's ideas of what he wants and how he would like his future to unfold differ from what are deemed by others as his best interests. The person may not want antibiotics, open heart surgery, kidney dialysis, a feeding tube, a tracheostomy, and so on. What the physicians or the family of a patient think is in the best interests of the patient may not be what the patient wants. Each of us has the right to refuse medical treatment, even if the treatment presumably will benefit us.

Who should be your HCP agent? It can be anyone you choose who is an adult and has the mental capacity to speak for you when you cannot. It can be a spouse, a brother or sister, a parent, a child, a friend. The important qualification is that they understand your values and wishes if you were to lose decisional capacity. The person must understand the rules. They should know that they are to make decisions for you when you cannot, and the decisions must be according to your values and wishes, not theirs. And you will want someone who, although they may love you and care for you very much, has the ability to make important decisions for you under what may be emotionally stressful circumstances.

The process of choosing and documenting your HCP agent varies from state to state, but generally it is simple. First, you must have sufficient mental capacity to understand what an HCP agent is and does. Then you choose your HCP agent and talk with that person, so they understand your wishes and know in which circumstance they may need to serve as HCP agent. An HCP form can be obtained from a hospital or physician or online from the department of health in your state.

The form is a legal document but does not require a lawyer to execute it. Some states require that the form be notarized. Other states do not have that requirement; you simply name your HCP agent, sign the form, and have your signature witnessed. Check on what the requirements of a witness are in your state. In the state of New York, where I live, witnesses must be 18 years or older and cannot be the HCP agent or alternate. Witnesses are asked to print and sign their name and to indicate the date and their address under the following statement: "I declare that the person who signed this document (meaning you, the person who is designating an HCP agent) is personally known to me and appears to be of sound mind and acting of his or her own free will. He or she signed (or asked another to sign for him or her) this document in my presence." It is important to date the form because if there are multiple HCP forms, the most recent one is valid. You can make as many copies of your HCP form as you like. You will want one for yourself and another for your HCP agent. You may want your physician to have one. Hospitals are required to ask if you have an HCP agent or other advance directive when you are admitted and, if you do not have an HCP agent, will encourage you to designate one and fill out a form.

Being an HCP agent and having financial or legal power of attorney are not the same. Although the HCP agent has broad powers in making health care decisions for you, appointing someone as your HCP agent does not give that person the right to pay your bills and take care of your legal affairs and, conversely, appointing someone who has power of attorney for you does not usually give that person the right to make health care decisions for you, unless that is stated explicitly. Appointing someone to have power of attorney for you often does require an attorney or must be arranged through your financial advisor. Of course, your HCP agent could also be the person who has power of attorney for you, but the two functions are different.

Although your HCP agent has the authority to make decisions for you, I do not advise HCP agents to behave in a preemptive or dictatorial fashion. They should talk with family members and other interested people to solicit their input and try to reach consensus on questions on which there may be disagreement. When family members continue to disagree, or there are questions that need clarification even when all agree, an ethics consultation may be helpful (see Chapter 4). The ethics consultant is someone who is experienced in end-of-life issues, as well as other problematic clinical situations, and may speak individually or collectively with family members, physicians, nurses, social workers, clergy, and others.

Sometimes a family meeting is useful. In a family meeting, relatives and perhaps close friends of the patient can discuss the important issues and questions with the attending physician and other relevant people, such as other physicians, nurses, social workers, a chaplain, and an ethics consultant. Family meetings may be convened by the attending physician, a social worker, a nurse, or an ethics consultant. During such meetings the medical team explains the clinical situation and its prognosis; the likely risks, benefits, and outcomes of various treatments; and the realistic goals of treatment. Family members and others are asked to express their views and concerns, which are addressed in an open, factual fashion. The person leading the meeting tries to reach consensus among family members about which treatments the patient should receive and which treatments should be withheld. If conflicts remain after all attempts have been made to reach consensus about what the patient would have wanted, then the HCP agent must decide.

So, in selecting an HCP agent, be sure to choose someone who:

1. understands that he or she is to make decisions for you when you are unable to make decisions for yourself;
2. knows your values and beliefs and wishes regarding end-of-life decisions;
3. understands that decisions are to be made according to your values, beliefs, and wishes, not those of the HCP;
4. is a person whom you trust and you think will be able to act rationally under emotionally stressful circumstances;
5. will talk with other family members, relevant friends, and health professionals to gather input in making important medical decisions.

Living Wills

A living will is a document that allows you to express, in as much detail as you want, your views and wishes about end-of-life situations that you think you could experience. Whereas HCP forms usually are brief, several pages at most, with limited space for you to explain your thoughts, a living will allows you to expand on your views and describe possible scenarios and how you would want to be treated in each of them. Templates and suggestions for living wills can be obtained at various websites simply by searching for living wills. Here are two examples, among many:

http://estate.findlaw.com/living-will/sample-living-will-form.
html

https://www.wikihow.com/Write-a-Living-Will

You can follow a suggested form, or you can make it up yourself, and your living will can be as terse or as expansive as you want.

You might say something like, "I wish to live and enjoy life as long as possible, but I do not wish to receive medical treatments that will only postpone the moment of my death from an incurable and terminal condition." Or conversely you might say, "I wish to live as long as possible, and I wish to receive all medical treatments that will preserve my life." You may want to anticipate situations in which you would want certain treatments to be withheld or applied. For example, you might say that, if you are in a coma for several weeks and there is no hope that your mental function would return, you would not want a permanent feeding tube or a tracheostomy. Or you could indicate your desire to receive such treatments under those conditions. Further, you might specify the circumstances under which you would want a Do Not Resuscitate (DNR) order to be written or not written. A DNR order means that you would not want your heart resuscitated if it stopped or had an ineffective rhythm. You may even want to be specific about what you mean by DNR. Narrowly, DNR may be interpreted to mean that the doctors would not compress your chest to revive your heart, but they may administer electric shocks or inject drugs. Broadly interpreted, DNR means you do not want anything done to resuscitate your heart if it stops working, including physical chest compressions, electric shocks, and drugs. Conversely, if you do want to receive certain treatments and make sure there is no mistake about avoiding or stopping them, you can be explicit about those wishes.

A living will also provides the opportunity to explain other details about how you would want to experience your last days. You may say that if at all possible you would want to die at home or in a specific location. You may attach other conditions or express the desire for certain experiences. Several years ago, during a course in which I was the facilitator for a small group of medical students, I assigned the students the task of creating a living will for themselves. One visionary student requested that his last days be spent in his kitchen, so he could enjoy the smells of food cooking and receive visitors there. He also, optimistically, asked that he be informed before he died that the Cubs had won the World Series . . . even if they had not.

You also may designate your HCP agent in your living will. Sometimes this is called a living will agent, but the functions and obligations are the same as an HCP agent. Thus, a living will can serve both as an HCP form and a vehicle for expressing your views about end-of-life matters.

Which Should I Do, Appoint an HCP Agent or Write a Living Will?

You should do one or the other, perhaps both. A living will allows you to expand on your thoughts and recite scenarios as examples of how you want decisions to be made for you. However, no matter how expansive and detailed your living will is, it is unlikely you will predict precisely the medical situations you will experience. In those situations, you want someone who knows your wishes to take into account the complexities of the circumstances as they are in the moment, not a theoretical situation that you tried to predict when you wrote your living will. Thus, you should appoint an HCP agent, either by executing an HCP form or by including the HCP agent in your living will.

Some people think—I am one of them—that a living will is unnecessary if you have an HCP agent who understands your values and wishes about end-of-life matters. In that case, what you would have written in a living will is understood fully by your HCP agent and thus a living will is not needed or may be confusing. The nuances of end-of-life decisions are complex, and your HCP agent should be able to navigate them as you would. Such an HCP agent might even sense when you might have changed your mind to seemingly contradict what you had expressed before you were ill. This should be very unusual, because your HCP agent is held to the high standard of representing your previously expressed wishes. But sometimes the clinical situation is very complex and there may be extenuating circumstances, such that you, if you could have made the decision yourself, might have done something contrary to your previously expressed wishes under those particular conditions. For example, if a person had expressed the wish to stop treatment and die, and then lost decisional capacity, an HCP agent might decide to continue treatment for a day or two longer until loved ones could arrive and be with that person before he died.

I said that I felt a living will was unnecessary for me because I have an HCP agent, my wife, who understands my wishes. This may seem to be a little cavalier on my part. It assumes that my HCP agent will be available when I need her. She may not be able to function as my HCP agent for the same reason I am not able to make my own decisions—accident, illness, or cognitive decline—or she may no longer be available for other reasons. You may want to anticipate this possibility by providing guidance to others who may be called on to make your decisions and appoint an alternate HCP agent (which I have done), create a living will, write another less formal statement, or simply have conversations with others you trust.

POLST—Physician's Orders for Life-Sustaining Treatment Forms

Many states provide a way to make your wishes known about end-of-life decisions through a special document called a POLST or Physician's Orders for Life-Sustaining Treatment form. In some states the document is called a MOLST (Medical Order for Life-Sustaining Treatment) form. A POLST or MOLST usually applies to people who are living at home or in a nursing or long-term care facility and who are expected to die within a year. The form is brief, brightly colored and thus highly visible, and is meant to guide caregivers and emergency personnel who may be called to your home or where you are living.

The POLST expresses your wishes with regard to certain end-of-life decisions, such as Do Not Resuscitate (DNR) orders and other life-sustaining treatments. For example, you can check a box that says you do want CPR (an attempt at cardiopulmonary resuscitation) or check a box that says you do not want resuscitation, but rather want a DNR order. You can indicate whether you do not want an endotracheal tube (DNI or Do Not Intubate order) or, instead, you do want a trial period of an endotracheal tube. You can designate whether you want limited medical interventions, unlimited interventions, or comfort care, meaning, you do not want medical interventions, but rather you simply want to be made comfortable. You can express your wishes with regard to the use of antibiotics, intravenous fluids, and feeding tubes and whether you want their use limited or not. The POLST form also can indicate what other advance directives you have, such as an HCP agent or a living will.

The POLST is a medical order, signed by a physician or medical professional and, in most states that have them, by the patient. It is meant to be a part of your medical record. It also should travel with you, meaning, if you are taken to a hospital from home or another facility, the POLST should accompany you. Some people keep the POLST form close to them. POLST forms have been observed to be taped inside the front door, to the refrigerator, or on the wall of a person's bedroom.

WHAT IF I DO NOT HAVE AN HCP AGENT, A LIVING WILL, OR A POLST? WHO WILL MAKE IMPORTANT HEALTH CARE DECISIONS FOR ME IF I AM UNABLE TO MAKE THEM?

All states in the United States have laws that describe who can make decisions for you when you become incapacitated and have not designated a surrogate decision-maker, although specifics and nomenclature vary.[1] I will use the state with which I am most familiar, New York, as an example. In New York, the Family Health Care Decisions Act identifies a priority list of people who may be asked to be your surrogate decision-maker, that is, someone who makes decisions for you. The list is as follows. Details may vary in other states.

1. Legally appointed guardian
2. Spouse or domestic partner
3. Adult child
4. Parent
5. Sibling
6. Close adult friend or relative who is familiar with the patient's views about health care

The first category is a court-appointed legal guardian. Although some people who have had decisional capacity and then lose it at the end of life have legal guardians, the second category, spouse or domestic partner, is usually the first relevant one. This means, in New York, that if a patient is not married but has a domestic partner, the domestic partner has the same authority as a spouse would have had.

The next category is an adult child, followed by a parent, then a sibling, and finally a close adult friend or relative who is familiar with the patient's views about health care. The law does not prescribe which child or parent or sibling should be selected, so it is not necessarily the oldest child or oldest sibling or one parent over the other. But it should be the person who is best able to represent the wishes of the patient.

This gives the attending physician both the responsibility and the latitude to designate as the surrogate decision-maker someone who seems best qualified to represent the wishes of the patient or, if the wishes are not known, at least to act in what are presumed to be the patient's best interests.

The final category is a close adult friend or relative who is familiar with the patient's views about health care. When all good faith efforts to locate a child or parent or brother or sister have failed—I have found that social workers, marvelous in so many ways, do an extraordinary job of locating hard to find children and siblings, sometimes at great distance—there may be other relatives or friends who know the patient well and understand their attitudes and wishes about end-of-life situations.

Usually there is agreement among family members about this process and what to do for the patient. Sometimes family members disagree. Disagreements may be about who will be the surrogate decision-maker or about other matters, and may arise from differences in values, religious views, past conflicts; from insufficient time to understand and assimilate the implications of the patient's condition; or simply when those involved have not had the opportunity to meet and discuss the medical facts and express their views to one another. The question is not what anyone else wants for the patient but what the patient would have wanted.

Everyone involved—family members, nurses, physicians, social workers, clergy—should try to reach a shared understanding of the patient's condition and what various treatments can and cannot accomplish. Although the surrogate decision-maker has the legal authority to make decisions for the patient, the attending physician should try hard to encourage interested parties to meet, discuss, and resolve differences. If differences cannot be resolved and it is important that decisions be made, the attending physician may rely on the surrogate decision-maker, according to the priority list in the law. A category cannot be skipped unless the person is not available or is unwilling to act as surrogate decision-maker. For example, if an adult child, a category which outranks siblings of the patient, is capable and willing to act as decision-maker, a brother or sister of the patient cannot be chosen to do that.

Of course, if an HCP agent has been identified and is available, the provisions of this law do not apply. Also, this law applies to individuals who have had the capacity to make decisions but lose it. Other laws provide for individuals who chronically or never had decisional capacity, such as the developmentally disabled or people who suffer from chronic mental disabilities.

IF THE LAW IN MY STATE DESIGNATES WHO SHOULD MAKE MY HEALTH CARE DECISIONS IF I HAVE NOT NAMED AN HCP AGENT, WHY SHOULD I GO TO THE TROUBLE OF PICKING AN HCP AGENT?

Naming an HCP agent assures that someone you trust and best knows your wishes will speak on your behalf to ensure that your preferences are followed if you are unable to express them. Leaving the designation of your surrogate decision-maker up to the law may result in having someone you do not want in that role. If you are worried that your HCP agent may become ill or otherwise is incapable of acting on your behalf, you may want to designate an alternative HCP agent who also understands your wishes, rather than leaving decision-making to the next person on a list.

WHAT IS THE ROLE OF THE LEGAL SYSTEM AND THE COURTS IN RESOLVING CONFLICTS AMONG FAMILY MEMBERS OR BETWEEN FAMILY AND THE MEDICAL STAFF?

Rarely, in highly contentious situations, the idea of seeking resolution in the courts comes up. The question may be about who should act as surrogate decision-maker. It may be about some other important decision in the management of the patient, such as disagreement on whether to continue kidney dialysis, a feeding tube, mechanical ventilation, and so on. The attending physician and those close to the patient should explore all means short of a court order, including conversations with individuals, family meetings, and ethics consultation. A court order may be detrimental because it can entrench the positions of those who disagree and generate a great deal of anger. However, if the family or the attending physician feels that all reasonable methods to achieve consensus have been exhausted and the patient's wishes or best interests are being subverted, they should consult with a lawyer or the legal staff of the hospital for advice about proceeding to seek a court order.

In the next chapter we will talk more about how conflicts that arise within families or between patients or families and health professionals in end-of-life situations may be resolved.

Chapter 4

RESOLVING ETHICAL CONFLICTS
The Role of Ethics Committees and Ethics Consultants

We repeat for the sake of emphasis and clarity that upon the concurrence of the guardian and family of Karen, should the responsible attending physicians conclude that there is no reasonable possibility of Karen's ever emerging from her present comatose condition to a cognitive, sapient state and that the life-support apparatus now being administered to Karen should be discontinued, they shall consult with the hospital "Ethics Committee" or like body of the institution in which Karen is then hospitalized. If that consultative body agrees . . . the present life-support system may be withdrawn and said action shall be without civil or criminal liability therefor, on the part of any participant, whether guardian, physician, hospital or others.

—In the Matter of Karen Quinlan, an Alleged Incompetent
Supreme Court of New Jersey, March 31, 1976

I n 1975, Karen Ann Quinlan, then age 21, reportedly consumed several alcoholic drinks and took Valium at a party after being on a diet and not eating much for several days. She complained of faintness and was taken home and put to bed. Fifteen minutes later her friends found she was not breathing. They took her to a hospital where she remained in a coma despite resuscitative efforts. Eventually she was deemed to be in a persistent vegetative state, with irreversible brain damage and intermittent respiratory failure, requiring a ventilator. She also received nourishment by nasogastric tube.

After several months, Karen's parents asked the hospital to stop the ventilator because they thought it was causing her to suffer more and was inappropriately prolonging her life. The hospital refused, fearing that the local prosecutor would charge the hospital with murder. Karen's parents brought suit to have the ventilator removed. This was denied initially but on appeal, the New Jersey Supreme Court, on March 31, 1976, granted their request. The Court said that her right to privacy included the right to decline treatment, her father could exercise this right for her, and the ventilator could be stopped if the family, the physicians, and an ethics committee agreed that she had no reasonable possibility of recovering cognition. Karen was taken off the ventilator but, contrary to expectation, she continued to breathe without the ventilator and lived another nine years, unconscious, bedridden, and fed artificially, until she died from respiratory failure in 1985.

This landmark decision was important because it was the first legal case in which the court recommended that hospitals should form ethics committees to resolve ethical questions related to the welfare and interests of patients. The usefulness of such committees became increasingly evident and more hospitals created them. Now the requirement that hospitals have an ethics committee or alternative means of addressing ethical questions, such as ethics consultants, is a feature of hospital accreditation.

The Quinlan decision also introduced the notion of advance directives, meaning, declaring in advance of developing various medical conditions what one's wishes might be in those situations or the appointment of a health care proxy (HCP) agent who can represent your wishes if you are unable to do so. We talked about advance directives in Chapter 3.

Another important case, that of Nancy Cruzan in 1990, shared many of the elements of the Karen Ann Quinlan situation. A major difference was that the Cruzan case rose to the United States Supreme Court, whereas the Quinlan case was decided by a state court, the New Jersey Supreme Court. In 1983 Nancy Cruzan, age 25, was involved in an automobile crash that left her in a persistent vegetative state. In 1986 her parents wanted to stop her feeding tube, but the hospital said it needed a court order to do so. The Missouri Supreme Court supported the decision to stop feeding her, but their decision was appealed to the U.S. Supreme Court, which in 1990 upheld the Missouri decision. In doing so, the court said that life-sustaining treatments may be withheld only if there was clear and convincing evidence that the patient would not want them. The court also affirmed that all of us have the right to refuse treatment and our family can exercise that right on our behalf if we are incapacitated. Later, a friend testified that Nancy had indicated that she would not want to live in the condition she was after the accident. A subsequent court order allowed life support to be removed and Nancy died 11 days later.

The Cruzan case established a precedent that was set by the highest court in the United States and affirmed both the importance of advance directives, such as a living will or instructions for a health care proxy agent, and the notion of having a surrogate decision-maker, someone who knows the wishes of the person, if the person is not capable of making his or her own decisions.

These two landmark cases made clear the importance of having an impartial means of navigating and deciding ethical questions that arise in health care, especially at the end of life, and they set the stage for the establishment of mechanisms to resolve ethical conflicts in hospitals and health care institutions, not only in the United States but elsewhere around the world.

HOW DOES AN ETHICS COMMITTEE WORK, WHAT DOES IT DO?

If you have never encountered an ethics committee, you may wonder what exactly it is and how it works. The term "ethics committee" sometimes is used in a general way to cover any mechanism that an institution uses to address ethical questions. The two most common are an ethics committee itself and an ethics consultation service. The hospital in which I work has both.

Our ethics committee is typical of committees in other institutions in the composition of its membership. It comprises about 20 people, including physicians, nurses, social workers, ethics consultants, a palliative care specialist, a hospital chaplain, administrators, a lawyer, and a person from the community outside the institution. The committee meets every one or two months.

The ethics committee's main tasks are twofold: (1) to create, review, and revise hospital policies that are relevant to ethical issues and (2) to develop educational programs and materials for hospital personnel and patients and families. Examples of policies that the ethics committee might develop are those that regulate Do Not Resuscitate orders, define the designation of decision-makers for patients who do not have them, protect patient privacy, stipulate the rights and responsibilities of patients, delineate procedures for donation of organs, and clarify conditions regarding medical students interacting with patients and learning from them.

During many meetings, in addition to fulfilling its policy and educational functions, the committee reviews a clinical case, not so much to provide guidance in real time for the patient and clinicians involved in the case, but to inform the committee members of the kinds of issues that are occurring in the hospital or to provide guidance to clinicians and hospital administrators on problematic ethical issues. For example, an ethics committee might consider how to deal with undocumented immigrants when they present to the emergency department in the face of the notion that they should be reported to authorities by emergency department personnel. Many hospitals have acknowledged that undocumented immigrants who are patients are fellow human beings in need of care; if health care facilities report them to authorities, that erodes the trust between the patient and health care provider and may deter the patient from seeking care. Another example is the question of prisoners' rights. Prisoners, although they relinquish many civil rights while incarcerated, retain most rights that relate to their own health and, like other patients, can make medical decisions for themselves, providing they have the mental capacity to do so.

HOW DO ETHICS CONSULTANTS HELP?

Because most ethical questions need attention quickly, they cannot wait for a meeting of the ethics committee. To convene a multi-member committee within the time that an ethical question needs to be addressed is impractical. Instead, these issues call for ethics consultants, individuals who are experienced in dealing with problematic situations that have ethical dimensions and can respond to requests in a timely manner.

Ethics consultants provide a nimbleness of response that is not possible with an ethics committee. Although ethics emergencies are unusual, the ethics consultants are available like other clinical consultants to respond within minutes to hours, as the case requires. Ethics consultants can be helpful to the patient, family, and clinicians by providing an additional experienced perspective and identifying the relevant ethical and practical issues, thus allowing the patient, family, and clinicians to focus on questions that have been defined better. Often, the ethics consultant's role resembles that of a mediator as well as an expert, helping to guide the hard decisions that families face and making sure they take into account advice from the medical team and make choices in line with their own values, especially those of the patient.

In our hospital, several people take turns responding to requests for ethics consultation, and they are identified on a published schedule that is available to everyone on the patient's clinical team. The ethics consultant reviews the patient's chart and other information and meets with the relevant people, such as the patient, family members, friends of the patient if necessary, and various health care professionals, including the attending physician, other physicians and nurses, social workers, and chaplains. Commonly the ethics consultant discusses the case with another colleague on the consultation service. The consultant places a note in the patient's chart, which summarizes the clinical features, identifies the ethical issues, some of which may not have been appreciated initially, and makes recommendations. Our ethics consultants respect the authority and responsibility of the attending physician, so they avoid making specific recommendations about medical care and try not to allow their own values to color their recommendations. Some recommendations, however, may be directive, such as to clarify the patient's wishes if the patient is able to express them, to identify a decision-maker if one is needed, to get social services involved to track down a relative, or to schedule a family meeting to discuss and resolve differences. If family meetings occur, they usually are led by the attending physician but may be led by a nurse or the ethics consultant. Our ethics consultants meet once a month to review all the cases of the previous month for the purposes of their own education and application of what they learn to the benefit of future patients, families, and health professionals.

WHO CAN REQUEST AN ETHICS CONSULTATION?

Typically, the attending physician asks for an ethics consultation, although others involved with the care of the patient may be empowered to do so. In my hospital, anyone directly involved in the clinical care of a patient—the patients themselves, family members, nurses, attending physicians, resident physicians in training, medical and nursing students, social workers, chaplains—may request an ethics consultation. Although we accept requests from any of the people mentioned, we encourage them to inform the attending physician that they are doing so, but we do not require it. In my experience, most ethics consultations are requested by the attending physician or on his or her behalf by a social worker or resident physician. A minority of consultations are requested by a patient or family member, but often when a health professional requests a consultation it is because of questions that have been brought up by the patient or family.

WHAT QUESTIONS MIGHT AN ETHICS CONSULTANT BE ASKED TO CONSIDER AND HOW CAN THE CONSULTATIONS BE USEFUL TO PATIENTS AND FAMILIES?

Questions arise constantly in the care of patients, both from the perspective of the patient and family and from the perspective of the physicians and clinical team. Usually the questions relate to clinical management: what diagnostic tests to order, which medications to prescribe, which procedures to perform. That is what medical practice is about and these questions usually are addressed in a straightforward manner by the clinicians caring for the patient. Sometimes, however, concerns about social, legal, or ethical matters may raise other questions. Also, the questions may not neatly sort out into medical, social, legal, or ethical categories, so it is not always clear whether there is an ethical issue. The person who poses the question—a patient, family member, physician, nurse, social worker—just wants advice about a complex and confusing situation, and they hope that the ethics consultant can help. I appreciate this and my approach as an ethics consultant is to respond and provide what perspective I can, without worrying whether the question is an ethical one.

The reasons for requesting ethics consultations are multiple and interrelated. A frequent one is to resolve disagreements among family members about medical decisions and other aspects of the care of a patient who cannot decide for himself. Sometimes members of the clinical team are concerned that an HCP agent seems to be acting contrary to the wishes of a patient. Or is the HCP agent coercing the patient in some way? In some cases, there may be questions about the ability of the HCP agent him- or herself to make decisions, particularly when the HCP agent has become ill or is failing mentally. Many requests ask for assistance in assessing the patient's ability to make decisions. Although the attending physician has the authority to decide whether the patient has decision-making capability, ethics consultants, because they have seen many patients with varying degrees of decision-making ability, can be helpful in advising about this. And, if the patient cannot make decisions, how do we determine what the patient would have wanted, if there is no HCP agent or the HCP agent does not know?

The following clinical stories, created from my experience, will give you a glimpse of the wide range of cases in which an ethics consultant can be helpful.

• Disagreement between siblings about the care of their father.

A social worker requested an ethics consultation because she saw that a patient's son and daughter disagreed strongly about whether a DNR order should be written for their father. The patient was a 69-year-old man who had been admitted to the hospital because of multiple fractures sustained during a motor vehicle accident. He had had coronary artery disease and chronic obstructive pulmonary disease for many years and had been treated for stomach cancer several years ago. On the second day after admission, he had a stroke, became semi-conscious, and lost the ability to communicate. Several days after that, he developed septicemia, a systemic infection that caused low blood pressure, requiring intravenous medications to maintain his blood pressure. Pneumonia ensued and, because he had difficulty breathing, a tube was passed through his mouth into his trachea—an endotracheal tube—and connected to a mechanical ventilator.

In view of the progressively declining likelihood that the patient would recover, the attending physician asked the family if they thought that the patient would have wanted a DNR order. The daughter said that her father had made it clear before he became ill that he wanted to be resuscitated if his heart stopped working. The son, who also was the patient's HCP agent, acknowledged that his father was a fighter. But now that he had had a stroke and septicemia and required medications to maintain his blood pressure and a ventilator to help him breathe, the son was convinced that his father would not want to be resuscitated to live in this condition or linger for months in a nursing home.

A family meeting was held that included the son and daughter, the attending physician, the social worker, several nurses, and the ethics consultant. Attempts to come to agreement initially were unsuccessful, but in a subsequent meeting after thorough review of the seriousness of the patient's condition and consideration that cardiac resuscitation would not likely to be successful in returning the patient to any meaningful life, the daughter agreed to a DNR order. The clinical team kept both daughter and son informed of the patient's condition. One week later the patient's heart developed ventricular fibrillation. He was not resuscitated and died.

- The HCP agent seems to be acting contrary to the wishes of the patient.

An intensive care physician became concerned that a patient's daughter, who also was the patient's HCP agent, wanted to do something that seemed contrary to the patient's previously expressed wishes. The patient was an 83-year-old woman who had been admitted several days before from a nursing home because of pulmonary edema (fluid in the lungs) and pneumonia. She had multiple medical conditions, including diabetes, hypertension, and atrial fibrillation. She also had become progressively demented and now, because of the dementia and the effects of her illness, she was unable to make decisions for herself.

About a year before, when she still had the mental capacity to do so, she had completed an HCP form, designating her daughter as her HCP agent. She also appended the statement, "If I become terminally ill or if I am unconscious with no hope of recovery, I do not want cardiac resuscitation, I do not want to be intubated, and I do not want a feeding tube." Now, she was in respiratory distress and having difficulty with her tracheal and oral secretions. The daughter learned that an endotracheal tube with mechanical ventilation could relieve her mother of her distress and told the physician that she wanted her mother to have that, but the physician thought this seemed contrary to what the patient wanted.

The ethics consultant spoke with the daughter who said that she and her mother had had explicit conversations about intubation. The daughter said that her mother told her that, although she was opposed to chronic intubation, she felt that, should the occasion arise, short-term intubation to relieve suffering or to treat a temporary condition would be permissible. The daughter felt that her mother would want short-term intubation now to relieve the suffering of her distressed breathing and avoid aspiration of secretions.

The intensive care physician and the daughter agreed to mechanical ventilation through an endotracheal tube for up to ten days. The tube would be discontinued sooner if the patient could breathe comfortably during trials without it, but after ten days it would be withdrawn if the patient had not improved. This plan was felt to be in accordance with the patient's wishes. After three days, the pneumonia and pulmonary edema improved, the patient was able to breathe without mechanical assistance, and the endotracheal tube was removed. She was discharged to her nursing home five days later.

- Is the patient being influenced by someone to act against her own wishes?

A 58-year-old woman had had surgery to remove a malignant brain tumor about a week before. The surgery itself had been long and her post-operative course was complicated by infection throughout her bloodstream, gastrointestinal bleeding, and clots in her leg veins, which led to pieces of clot traveling to her lungs to create pulmonary emboli. She required mechanical ventilation through a tracheostomy and was being fed via a tube through her abdominal wall into her stomach. She seemed alert and able to understand questions, but she could not speak because of the tracheostomy. She mouthed her answers to questions, pointed to letters on a printed alphabet, and raised her eyes up to indicate "yes" and down for "no."

The patient had stated in a living will, executed five years previously, that if she had an incurable or irreversible condition, she would not want life-sustaining treatment. When the attending physician and the nurses spoke with her about continuing treatment options, she expressed the wish to die. However, the patient's daughter, who was her HCP agent, wanted her mother to live and, when the daughter visited, encouraged her mother to continue whatever treatments were available. Indeed, after visits by the daughter, the patient seemed to reverse her views on dying and indicated that she wanted to continue to live. Thus, the patient vacillated between asking her caregivers to stop life-sustaining treatments and asking that they continue them.

The ethics consultant met separately with the patient, the daughter, and the physician. The consultant agreed with the attending physician that the patient had the capacity to make her own decisions. Thus, the daughter could not make decisions for her mother as HCP agent, because her mother still possessed decisional capacity. Of course, the daughter could influence her mother simply because of her relationship and concern. The consultant also pointed out that sometimes people are ambivalent about their situation when they are very sick. The ethics consultant then met with the patient, her daughter, and the attending physician together. They agreed to continue current treatments and review the situation in one week. The patient improved and was discharged to home care, then to hospice care at home. She died two months later.

- Does the HCP agent have the capability to act as an HCP agent?

A 42-year-old woman suffered a traumatic brain injury when she fell as she was climbing a mountain. She was transported to a trauma center where a CT scan showed a large intracranial hemorrhage. She underwent surgery to relieve the pressure from the bleeding. Postoperatively she suffered a seizure. She was sedated and placed on mechanical ventilation. The clinical team anticipated that several decisions would need to be made soon, such as whether to insert a feeding tube into the stomach and, in a week or two, whether to convert the endotracheal tube to a permanent tracheostomy. Perhaps at some point a DNR order would need to be considered.

The patient's father, age 78, was her HCP agent. However, family members had noted a decline in his mental abilities. He sometimes appeared confused and forgetful. The patient's sister felt that she was better able to make decisions for the patient than their father. Another sibling, a brother of the patient, agreed that the father should relinquish his duties as HCP agent, and the wife of the father, who was the mother of the three siblings, also agreed. However, when the father was asked to do that, he said that he was still capable of making decisions for his daughter. The ethics consultant and the attending physician met with the father. The attending physician, with input from the ethics consultant, determined that, although the father was forgetful and a little slow mentally, he had the capacity to understand the facts of his daughter's condition, her prognosis, and the risks and benefits of various treatments. During a subsequent family meeting, all agreed that the father should continue as HCP agent, but he would discuss medical decisions on behalf of the patient with his wife and the patient's siblings and solicit their input.

If the attending physician had determined that the father was not capable of functioning as the HCP agent, the physician could recognize another person, presumably one of the patient's siblings, to act as surrogate decision-maker for the patient. The process of doing this may vary from one state to another. You may want to refresh your understanding of this by returning to Chapter 3 where we talked about advance directives and what to do when someone has not been designated or is not available to make decisions for us when we cannot make our own decisions.

- Can surgeons do a medically indicated operation in a patient who cannot give consent when no one is available to speak for the patient? This is an example of the kind of consultation that is more urgent than most.

An 82-year-old man had three days of abdominal and back pain and went to the emergency department of his local hospital. A CT scan showed a leaking abdominal aortic aneurysm. He was alert and able to give consent for surgery and the aneurysm was repaired by sewing a graft at the site of the aneurysm in the abdominal aorta.

After surgery, the man was admitted to the intensive care unit, where he was sedated. The next day he passed large amounts of blood from his rectum. Colonoscopy showed ischemic colitis, a condition that results from insufficient blood to the lining of the colon and causes bleeding. This is a recognized complication of aortic aneurysm repair in some patients because a major artery to the colon must be removed when the graft is placed to repair the aneurysm. The surgeons advised an immediate operation to remove the ischemic portion of colon that was deprived of its blood supply and thus no longer had oxygen. Because of sedation, the patient was unable to give consent for the second surgery and he had no HCP agent. A brother in a distant state was contacted but said he did not want to be involved. Attempts to contact other relatives were unsuccessful. What should the surgeons do? Should they continue to try to contact someone who could act as surrogate decision-maker for the patient? Should they wait several hours until the patient would be less sedated and perhaps able to understand sufficiently to consent to surgery? Or should they go ahead and perform the surgery without explicit permission from the patient or a surrogate decision-maker?

In this situation, the ethics consultant advised the surgeons to do what was medically indicated in the best interest of the patient. In the absence of evidence that the patient would not have wanted the operation, it should be done. Physicians are justified in providing emergency and urgent care when patients need it but are unable to give consent. This, of course, happens routinely in emergency departments and elsewhere when urgent situations need to be addressed in patients who are unable to give consent and no one is available to speak for them. That is simply good medical practice.

In this chapter we considered what might be done to mediate and resolve ethical questions that arise in the course of end-of-life experiences, questions that patients and families have as well as physicians and other health care givers. Sometimes, dying people reach a point where there is nothing else to do to treat the underlying disease process, whether they or their loved ones continue to have questions or not. What are the options then? In the next two chapters we will review how treatment in these situations can shift to so-called comfort care and its variations, and then we will consider options for taking your own life, if you are so inclined.

Chapter 5
PALLIATIVE CARE

"I am delightfully unwell."

—Woman in hospice care

I met Troy[1] in his hospital room about three months after his brain surgery. Troy had been well for most of his 56 years, except for the usual childhood diseases and sports injuries. Several months before his surgery, he had developed headaches and, while on the job as a maintenance worker at the county office building, he had suffered a seizure. By the time the emergency medical technicians (EMTs) arrived, Troy had regained consciousness. The EMTs took him to the hospital emergency department (ED), where his wife Shawna met him.

After initial evaluation in the ED, Troy was admitted to the hospital. A cluster of medical tests, including a brain scan, identified a tumor, which was diagnosed as a meningioma. Most meningiomas are benign, meaning that their cells do not show the typical aggressive growth of a cancer, but some are malignant. Regardless, meningiomas almost always occur in the brain, so any growth, benign or malignant, can cause symptoms and affect important brain functions. In Troy's case, the meningioma clearly seemed to be the culprit with regard to the headaches and seizure. Troy needed brain surgery.

Troy's tumor turned out to be malignant and the surgeons were not able to remove it completely.

His post-operative course was complicated by the buildup of fluid in the cavities of his brain, which required the insertion of a tube into the cavities to drain the fluid. Troy recovered sufficiently to return home, hoping to improve further so that he could receive other forms of treatment, perhaps radiation or chemotherapy.

About a month and a half after his surgery, while at home, Troy experienced sudden sharp pain in his chest and coughed up some blood. Shawna rushed him to the hospital where an ED physician diagnosed a pulmonary embolus. This was attributed to a small piece of coagulated blood that had traveled to his lungs from a clot in his lower right leg.

In the intensive care unit, Troy developed pneumonia and, because of the great difficulty he had breathing, his doctors inserted an endotracheal tube, a tube that goes through the nose or mouth into the trachea, and connected it to a mechanical ventilator. From time to time the doctors tried having Troy breathe without the assistance of the ventilator, but he could not, so it became evident that he would need long-term breathing assistance. An endotracheal tube causes irritation of the trachea when it is in place a long time, so after about ten days

Troy's medical team removed the endotracheal tube and replaced it with a surgical tracheostomy, to which they attached the ventilator.

Because Troy was unable to swallow liquids or food, he received fluids and some nourishment intravenously. This became insufficient to meet his nutritional requirements, so his doctors inserted a tube called a PEG (percutaneous endoscopic gastrostomy) surgically into his stomach to provide calories and nourishment. Other complications arose. Troy's blood became infected with bacteria, which required antibiotics. He also began to bleed slowly from his gastrointestinal tract, perhaps related to the blood thinners he received to prevent further clots from going to his lungs or brain. A urinary tract infection developed, requiring more antibiotics. A brain scan showed that the remaining tumor was getting larger.

At each step of this horrible, complicated course, Troy and Shawna conferred with the doctors and nurses to discuss what was happening and what the particular interventions—the drainage tube in the cavities of his brain, mechanical breathing assistance, tracheostomy, PEG, antibiotics, and so on—were intended to do and what side effects they might expect. Although he was lightly sedated, Troy remained aware of his condition. He was not able to speak because of the tracheostomy, which prevented air from passing through his vocal cords, but he was able to communicate with Shawna, his sons Jeremy and Simon, friends who visited, and the hospital team by writing on a pad, pointing to letters on a printed alphabet, mouthing his words, or making eye and facial movements. He retained full mental capacity to make medical decisions.

About six weeks into this second hospitalization, Ruby, a nurse practitioner on the clinical team caring for Troy, asked me to get involved as an ethics consultant. It was now three months after the surgery to remove, incompletely, the malignant meningioma. Ruby told me that Troy had recently begun to express his wish to die, and she and others caring for him were concerned whether those expressions were his true wishes. Could I speak with Troy and Shawna and help sort this out?

When I walked into Troy's room, Shawna was with him, sitting in a chair, reading a magazine. Troy was in his bed. The ventilator had been disconnected temporarily and Troy seemed to be breathing well without it. I could see several other tubes leading into or out of his body—an intravenous line in his left arm, another intravenous line called a PICC (peripherally inserted central catheter) in his right arm, the PEG feeding tube, and the clear plastic bag that was connected to his urinary catheter.

I introduced myself to Troy and Shawna and explained that I was a member of the ethics consultation team. I told them I had been asked to help in the management of Troy's complicated course. I stated that the nurses and doctors who had been caring for Troy and who had been so close to both Troy and Shawna over the past several weeks had wondered whether Troy's wishes about his treatment had changed. I listened to what Shawna told me. It was clear that she spoke for Troy. Troy was not able to speak because of the tracheostomy, but from time to time he would nod and otherwise signal that he agreed with her. This is what they told me.

From the beginning, from the time that Troy suffered his seizure and they learned the news that the meningioma was malignant, Troy and Shawna hoped, along with the physicians and nurses, that he could recover sufficiently for him to consider further treatment with radiation or chemotherapy. And, as each complication developed—the pulmonary embolus, the need for mechanical breathing assistance, the insertion of the PEG tube and other invasions, the bacteria in the blood, the urinary tract infection—they shared an optimism that it could be remedied, and he could recover. But as each piece of bad news sunk in, they slowly realized the gravity of their situation and what it probably meant for Troy. The tumor that remained in Troy's brain was still growing, and, just yesterday, his kidneys had begun to fail, which meant he would need kidney dialysis. Their optimism became tempered by an increasing grasp on reality—Troy probably would not survive this.

Troy had appointed Shawna to be his health care proxy (HCP) agent at the beginning of the first hospitalization three months ago. They had talked even before that about their views on end-of-life decisions. During the first hospitalization it was difficult for them to speak openly about the possibility that Troy might die, but now Troy brought it up. They realized that Troy's medical condition was futile, meaning, nothing could be done to reverse the inexorable course of his underlying disease, the growth and spread of the meningioma. Yes, some of the complications—the pneumonia and subsequent ventilation with a machine, the inability to eat, the infections of his blood and urinary tract, and now the failure of his kidneys—could be treated and perhaps temporarily improved. But he and Shawna realized that nothing was going to restore him to anything close to his former health and that, in fact, he was dying. They talked about this with their sons Jeremy and Simon. Together, Troy and his family felt that they wanted Troy home.

We asked the Palliative Care team to see Troy. They helped the hospital clinical team shift from the intensive, aggressive care, which had been characteristic of Troy's in-hospital treatment until that time, to comfort care, which, as we will see, is not cessation of care but a different kind of care, with its own set of plans and objectives. The social worker on the clinical team arranged a schedule of visiting nurses and aides to help care for Troy at home. Troy seemed to be able now to breathe sufficiently well without the ventilator. The nurses instructed Shawna in how to use and maintain the PEG, and Troy went home. A hospice nurse visited him daily. Troy died of complications of pneumonia three weeks later, after falling into a coma, in the company of Shawna and his sons.

WHAT IS PALLIATIVE CARE?

For patients like Troy, palliative care is an appropriate option at the end of life. Millions of patients and their families choose palliative care every year. So, what does palliative care mean and what does it entail?

Palliative care focuses on the comfort of the patient. It is interdisciplinary and may include physicians, nurses, social workers, chaplains, and other professionals. The goals of palliative care are to prevent and relieve suffering, to support as normal a life as possible, and to improve quality of life. It is not aimed at cure or reversal of the disease. Palliative care applies not only to people with terminal cancer but also to individuals with other fatal disorders, such as terminal lung, heart, kidney, and neurological diseases.

In an end-of-life setting, palliative care usually comes after care that has focused on the diagnosis and treatment of one's medical condition. That care can be aggressive and seeks to contain or reverse the cause of the illness that is leading to death. Patients and families generally choose palliative care when it becomes evident that treatments of the fatal disorder are ineffective or futile, that is, no treatment will result in meaningful improvement of the patient's medical condition. Sometimes patients say they have "had enough" and simply want to be allowed to die as comfortably as possible. Patients and loved ones accept that the patient will die soon regardless of treatments aimed at the underlying disease. Most people in such a situation want to remain comfortable among loved ones, in familiar surroundings, and attended by appropriate health care professionals. Palliative care seeks to do just that.

One could make a good argument that elements of palliative care apply to the care of all patients, whether they are at the end of life or not, and ensure that every patient is as comfortable as possible. So palliative care is a shift in emphasis; it does not mean that a patient, her family, and the medical team are "giving up" on the patient. Instead, it is a different kind of care—a kind that still requires planning and understanding of what may be accomplished. All care, but especially comfort care at the end of life, should align with the wishes of the patient.

People sometimes confuse the terms "palliative care" and "hospice." Hospice, as it applies currently in the United States, is a form of palliative care for people whose life expectancy is estimated to be less than six months. Hospice care typically is contracted through an agency that specializes in it and usually occurs outside the hospital wherever the patient is living—at home, in a nursing home, in an assisted living facility—although sometimes it occurs in an in-patient hospital unit.

In Chapter 1, I said that one of the differences in dying now compared to the past is the increase in medical expenditures at the end of life. Does hospice or palliative care save money? One study of Medicare costs for providing hospice care in nursing homes showed that, although hospice care has grown for nursing home residents and was associated with less aggressive care near death, overall Medicare expenditures in the last year of life increased.[2] Spending on hospice care was greater but costs of hospital or other care did not diminish. The study attributed the higher hospice expenditures in part to an increased usage of hospice care and longer treatment under hospice, largely because of the growth in number of nursing home hospice residents with non-cancerous diseases, such as terminal lung, heart, kidney, and neurological diseases. Should we be disturbed by this? I don't think so. It seems appropriate to expand hospice treatment to include conditions other than cancer and to make people more comfortable and improve the quality of life as they are dying. If that costs more, I am willing to accept it.

DO NOT RESUSCITATE (DNR) AND DO NOT INTUBATE (DNI) ORDERS DURING PALLIATIVE CARE

You may decide to allow your physician to write orders that instruct your caregivers not to resuscitate your heart if it stops functioning (a DNR order) or not to insert a tube into your trachea, an endotracheal tube, to assist breathing (DNI). We talked about this in Chapter 3 in the context of making our wishes known in advance about end-of-life decisions. You may feel that under the circumstances of your illness, if your heart stops or your lungs have reached a point of extreme dysfunction, you would not want to continue to live after cardiac resuscitation or with a tube in your trachea. Sometimes, people who make these decisions reason that these events are a signal that it is time to die. DNR and DNI orders are not limited to people who are undergoing palliative care. People with many acute and chronic conditions or people who anticipate having those conditions someday may consider DNR or DNI or both. A person might simply say, for many reasons, something like, "If my heart stops, I do not want to be resuscitated." Or, "If my breathing and lung function are so bad that an endotracheal tube is recommended, I don't want it."

DNR and DNI orders are independent, that is, a person might choose one without the other. Before a physician writes either a DNR or DNI order, the physician and the patient should talk about the intent and possible consequences of "being DNR or DNI." If the patient is unable to have such a conversation or make a decision about such an order, the conversation should be with the patient's HCP agent or other surrogate decision-maker.

With regard to a DNR order, the discussion should include an explanation of what it means for a heart to stop, what it means to resuscitate it, and what the likely outcomes might be after attempts at resuscitation. When a heart stops working, usually it is because of a serious arrhythmia, such as ventricular fibrillation, which may or may not be responsive to electric shocks or medications. The discussion should be clear about what resuscitation means. Some patients do not like the idea of compressing their chest, which can be rigorous and may break ribs, but they may accept administration of electric shocks or drugs that are intended to restore normal heart rhythm. Broadly interpreted, DNR means you do not want anything done to resuscitate your heart if it stops, including physical chest compressions, electric shocks, and drugs that stimulate the heart. You or your decision-maker should understand what DNR means before you decide for or against a DNR order.

The discussion also should be factual about the expected outcome of cardiac resuscitation. People may be conditioned to have unrealistic expectations of the success of cardiac resuscitation by what they see on television dramas, which usually depict a high rate of recovery after cardiac resuscitation. In real life, fewer than 20% of patients who are resuscitated in a hospital survive to leave the hospital and those who are discharged often have significant mental and medical deterioration.

Similar honest discussions should occur when a person contemplates implementing a DNI order. You should talk about the circumstances that might lead to consideration of an endotracheal tube. Such tubes usually are connected to a mechanical ventilator. What are the implications of that? You should understand that the duration of treatment with an endotracheal tube is limited to about two weeks because of the tissue reaction within the trachea that occurs over that time. If mechanical ventilation is to continue, the endotracheal tube usually will need to be replaced by a tracheostomy, which is a direct, surgically created communication through the front of the neck to the trachea, with its own set of complications over the long term. Patients or their surrogates should consider in advance what will happen when an endotracheal tube has reached the end of its usefulness. Will they be willing to allow the medical team to convert the endotracheal tube to a permanent tracheostomy or should they withdraw the endotracheal tube, stop mechanical ventilation, and thus, most likely, allow the person to die?

It can be very difficult to discuss the medical details of your or your loved one's possible death, but being careful, specific, and thorough in these discussions and consequent decisions will ensure that you have a firm plan that everyone understands as you prepare for the uncertainties that lie ahead.

TREATMENT OF ACUTE CONDITIONS DURING PALLIATIVE CARE

A common misconception about palliative care is that acute conditions that arise during the patient's terminal course may not be treated. It is not the case that these conditions are neglected. On the contrary, since the main purpose of palliative care is to keep the person comfortable, it is appropriate under some circumstances to treat acute conditions, such as pain, difficulty breathing, and anxiety. Consider the following story.

Mel is a 78-year-old man with advanced lung cancer, who accepts that he probably has less than six months to live. He spends most of his time at home with his wife, Sarah, who is his HCP agent. Mel has received palliative care at home through a local hospice for the past two months. His pain is largely controlled by naproxen, a common over-the-counter pain reliever. He feels that he has an acceptable quality of life. He enjoys visits from his children, grandchildren, and friends, and sometimes he is able to go shopping with Sarah. One morning Mel is awakened by nausea and suddenly vomits a large amount of blood. Sarah takes him to the hospital ED where an upper gastrointestinal endoscopy, an examination of the esophagus, stomach, and upper small intestine, reveals a bleeding ulcer, which is cauterized through the endoscope to stop the bleeding. A side effect of naproxen is gastrointestinal bleeding and the doctors think that may be the problem now. After the ED team stabilizes Mel, they admit him to the intensive care unit (ICU), where his treatment includes placing a nasogastric (NG) tube through his nose into his stomach, giving him anti-ulcer medications, and, of course, stopping the naproxen.

Here are some questions you might have about Mel's initial treatment. As you take into account your own values and views about his medical situation, do you think Sarah should have taken him to the ED in the first place? After he arrived at the ED, should he have had endoscopy? How about the NG tube? Should he have been admitted to the ICU? These questions might arise from a belief that treatment of acute conditions is a departure from the treatment of a dying patient, particularly because some of the treatments are invasive and uncomfortable, such as endoscopy and the NG tube. But many patients and physicians would say that the relief of discomfort and the resolution of acute, limited conditions that cause discomfort and suffering are appropriate in the course of palliative care. In Mel's situation, the ED physicians did not know what was causing the acute bleeding, but it seemed reasonable to do a diagnostic test, in this case endoscopy, to try to find out the cause and treat it if possible. The intent here, in the name of comfort care, was to reverse the acute condition, which was causing such distress for Mel, while acknowledging that the underlying cancerous process that is leading to his death would not be improved. Even during comfort care, some discomfort may be tolerated to achieve relief of the acute condition, meaning, although doing endoscopy and passing an NG tube may be temporarily uncomfortable for Mel, there is a good likelihood that they will lead to improvement of his acute condition and thus allow Mel to be more comfortable.

Let's carry Mel's story a step or two further. On the second day in the ICU, he develops shortness of breath and coughing. A chest X-ray and sputum examination confirm a diagnosis of pneumonia. The pneumonia worsens over several days with the consequence that Mel has trouble breathing, he seems to gasp for air. The ICU doctors propose inserting an endotracheal tube and connecting it to a mechanical ventilator to help him breathe easier. If you were Mel, what would you want? Suppose Mel becomes confused and loses his capacity to make decisions. Does that affect your views about what should be done now? Of course, Sarah, as his HCP agent, will now begin to make these decisions for him. What do you think she should do? Somewhere along the course of Mel's hospitalization, someone may have suggested a DNR order. Should that have been written earlier when the diagnosis of disseminated cancer was first made, or later when Mel was admitted to the ICU, or now?

How you answer these additional questions might depend on how you reconcile some competing considerations. First, you may want to make Mel more comfortable, which is the intention of the endotracheal tube and mechanical assistance by the ventilator. But you also may acknowledge that, at some time during the course of his decline, inevitably he will experience something like this as the prelude to his death—perhaps pneumonia, kidney failure, or a cardiac arrhythmia that results in ineffective heart action. You might say, "Yes, we will insert an endotracheal tube to relieve his distress, but the endotracheal tube cannot be left in place indefinitely." After a couple of weeks, the endotracheal tube will need to be replaced by a permanent tracheostomy, if the treatment plan is to continue to provide mechanical ventilation for Mel. This raises the difficult question, "Are we willing to stop an intervention after we have started it?" In this case, before the decision to insert the endotracheal tube is made, Mel, or Sarah his HCP agent, and the medical team should have a discussion about how the future might unfold as regards the endotracheal tube. One outcome could be that the pneumonia resolves, and Mel does not need the endotracheal tube and it can be withdrawn. Another outcome could be that the endotracheal intubation is not successful, and Mel and his family are confronted with whether they should allow the medical team to convert the endotracheal tube to a permanent tracheostomy or whether they should withdraw the endotracheal tube and allow him to die.

A PERSPECTIVE ON PALLIATIVE CARE

I re-emphasize that palliative care is not cessation of care, but rather a different kind of care that requires planning, with understanding of what may be accomplished, all consistent with the wishes of the patient, expressed by him or his surrogate. One should consider the symptoms and complications that may need attention in a dying person—pain, difficulty breathing, coughing, excessive secretions in the mouth and throat, nausea and vomiting, constipation, poor appetite, weight loss, anxiety.[3,4] Generally, patients and their loved ones want these conditions to be taken care of, because they want the patient to be comfortable and it is distressing to experience them, both as a patient and as a loved one. But they also may acknowledge limits in the treatment of them. Sometimes the treatment of an acute condition just delays an inevitable, imminent death. The patient and family may realize that the acute condition, such as pneumonia, untreated, may be an appropriate means to hasten death, and they accept that now is the time to die.

Also, a common concern of friends and loved ones of a dying person is that the person does not want to eat. We feel that to eat is to be well, so we want the person to eat. It is important to appreciate that as death approaches, the desire to eat diminishes. That is normal. Physicians, nurses, and loved ones need to decide when to encourage the dying patient to eat and when to accept that not eating is part of the natural process of dying.

In the United States, Great Britain, and increasingly in other countries, the use of palliative care has grown in recent decades as more patients, families, and medical professionals become aware of its applications. Indeed, in the United States, over the past decade, palliative care programs have increased by more than 150%; almost 90% of hospitals with over 300 beds and most hospitals with over 50 beds have palliative care programs.[2]

Most people do not specifically anticipate the use of palliative care in their advance directives. However, when the time comes to make a decision about palliative care, it appears consistent with the views and values of many people as they have previously expressed them, so to shift from acute care to palliative care seems natural.

In the first chapter, we looked at the many ways that the process of dying has changed, including interventions that people might view as interfering with a "good death," such as not dying at home, but rather in an acute care facility; being treated with potent medications and high-tech gadgetry; and sometimes being separated from loved ones and familiar surroundings. Does palliative care help take us back to the good death? I believe it is a move in the right direction. We cannot return to yesteryear, of course. The current technology that is associated with such vexing complications for some of us at the end of life also brings much benefit to many others. But whatever we can do to maintain human dignity and preserve the satisfaction of human relationships, seems right.

Whether one chooses palliative care or not as death approaches, the dying process unfolds pretty much according to natural processes. Some people, however, anticipating that death is imminent and inevitable, decide to take more explicit control of their dying and initiate actions to kill themselves. This is what we will talk about in the next chapter.

Chapter 6
MAY I CHOOSE TO KILL MYSELF?

Death is nature's remedy for all things.
—Charles Dickens, *A Tale of Two Cities*, Book 2, Chapter 1

Brittany Maynard received the bad news on New Year's Day 2014. She learned that she had brain cancer. It was an astrocytoma, a malignancy that carries a dismal prognosis. She was 29, recently married, and well educated, having earned a bachelor's degree in psychology from the University of California Berkeley and a master's degree in education from the University of California Irvine. She had traveled widely in Asia and South America, teaching in orphanages in some of the places she visited. Brittany was, as the adage goes, "full of life" and she seemed ready for more of it.

Surgeons removed Brittany's tumor, but it recurred soon and progressed rapidly. In April 2014 she moved with her husband from California to Oregon so she could take advantage of Oregon's Death with Dignity Act, a law that allows people with terminal illnesses under specified conditions to take their own lives. At the time, California had no such law. Brittany's youth, attractiveness, and plight excited the interest of the public. She became an advocate for end-of-life rights and Death with Dignity laws. She was interviewed by national media and millions looked at her video on YouTube. Under the provisions of the Oregon law, Brittany obtained a prescription for a lethal dose of an oral barbiturate. On November 1, 2014, ten months after she learned her diagnosis, she swallowed the pills and died.[1]

Brittany Maynard's situation, somewhat atypical compared to the majority of people with a terminal illness largely because of the public nature of it, nevertheless shared many characteristics with others who are enduring the threats and debilitations of a terminal illness and who desire to take control over the time, circumstances, and other particulars of their death.

PHYSICIAN-ASSISTED DEATH

People use several terms to talk about taking one's own life with the help of a physician when one is terminally ill. Often this act is called physician-assisted suicide, sometimes physician-assisted death, or simply, assisted death. Some people object to calling such a death a suicide because, although a person does take explicit steps to kill him- or herself, the circumstances of the death are different than most suicides. This means that death would have arrived soon regardless of any action by the person, so the person's action simply hastens an imminent, inevitable death. Also, avoiding the term suicide seems to lessen the social stigma that is associated with that. For these reasons, I prefer the term physician-assisted death.

Laws that permit a physician to prescribe lethal medications to eligible patients have been called Death with Dignity laws. Such laws currently exist in several states—Oregon, since 1994; Washington, 2008; Vermont, 2013; California, 2015; Colorado, 2016; and Hawaii, 2019—and the District of Columbia, since 2017. Montana, by decision of the state Supreme Court in 2009, also permits physician-assisted death under conditions similar to those described by state laws elsewhere. Proposals to enact Death with Dignity laws in other states currently are under consideration. Several states have rejected such proposals in recent years.

Canada, by decision of its Supreme Court in February 2015, became the first country that has a common law system to legalize physician-assisted death. Under common law, legal processes may be developed by the courts through precedents and case decisions. Physician-assisted death already is legal in several other countries, including Belgium, The Netherlands, Luxemburg, and Switzerland, but is illegal in the United Kingdom.

Not surprisingly, Death with Dignity laws are highly controversial. Advocates claim that for people with terminal illnesses, who may suffer unbearable pain, have no interest in eating, experience severe limitations in ability to move and care for themselves, or feel a profound loss of dignity, the legal option to kill themselves in a non-traumatic, perhaps even comfortable way can be liberating and fulfills notions of mercy and quality of life. And it seems to align with the fundamental principle in medicine: promotion of the welfare of the patient. Perhaps most important, it gives the person more autonomy to control circumstances that seem to have gotten out of control.

Opponents advance several arguments, the principal one being that taking one's own life is immoral. This is the position of some religious groups, but one does not have to be a religious person to object on moral grounds. There are other ways, opponents say, rather than taking one's own life, to deal with the pain and debility of terminal illness. Some people also feel that the involvement of a physician violates the trust that people put in physicians; is my doctor trying to keep me alive or kill me? Further, although current laws stipulate that the person who desires to kill him- or herself must have the mental capacity to make that decision, and the decision cannot be made by another person on their behalf, advocates for vulnerable people, including not only the mentally disabled but also the poor, elderly, uneducated, or physically disabled, warn that such laws could be abused or modified and start us down the "slippery slope" of ridding society of people who may be perceived as undesirable.

The name itself, Death with Dignity, is viewed in different ways. Proponents see the grave indignities that may accompany the dying process, such as loss of control over one's body, unrelenting pain, debility, and the consequences of various intubations and procedures, and believe that such laws allow the dying person to preserve some dignity by terminating his or her life in a painless, controlled manner. Critics as well as sympathizers point out that all dying, whether by one's own actions or not, should be managed with attention to the dignity of the dying person.

Physicians also are conflicted. My physician's oath obligates me to the primacy of the welfare of the patient. How does that apply here? Is it in the interest of the welfare of my patient that I provide a means for her to escape her suffering and die? Am I abandoning her if I do not help her die? Or is the welfare of my patient best served by resisting dying? Some physicians say, "My commitment is to treat illness and preserve life, not to kill people." Along with some patients, physicians also sometimes worry that the trusting relationship with patients will be eroded.

Under existing state laws that permit physician-assisted death, physicians may choose whether to participate, meaning, whether to welcome and evaluate patients who seek a lethal medication and prescribe it for them. Many physicians who say they themselves would not participate, however, indicate they would be willing to refer a patient who requested a life-ending drug to another physician who had agreed to participate.

OREGON DEATH WITH DIGNITY LAW

The Oregon Death with Dignity Act, which has been a model for laws in other states and can be taken as typical of them, specifies several requirements that must be met before a prescription for a lethal drug may be prescribed.[2]

- The requesting patient must be 18 years of age or older and a resident of the state.
- The patient must make two oral requests to his or her physician separated by at least fifteen days.
- The patient then must provide a written request on a specified form to the physician, signed in the presence of two witnesses. The witnesses, by signing the form, attest that the patient is known personally to them, has provided proof of identity, appears to be of sound mind, is not requesting the medication under duress or undue influence, and is not a patient of one or the other witness (if a witness is a health care professional). One witness shall not be a relative of the requester by blood or marriage or adoption, shall not be entitled to any portion of the requester's estate after death, and shall not be associated with the health care facility where the requester is a patient or resident.
- The diagnosis and prognosis of death within six months must be confirmed by both the prescribing physician and another physician.
- Both physicians also must determine whether the patient has the mental capability to make the decision to request a lethal drug.
- If either physician believes that the patient's judgment is impaired by a mental disorder, the patient must be referred for a psychological examination.

- The prescribing physician must inform the patient of alternatives to the Death with Dignity Act, including comfort care, hospice care, and pain control.
- The prescribing physician must ask the patient to notify his or her next of kin about the request for a lethal drug, but the patient is not obligated to comply.
- Prescribing physicians must report to state authorities all prescriptions they write for lethal medications. Reporting is not required if a patient begins the request process but does not actually receive a prescription.

The Act prohibits euthanasia, meaning, a physician or other person cannot directly administer a medication to end a person's life. It states that physicians, other health care personnel, and health systems are not obligated to participate. And it stipulates that ending one's life in accordance with the law does not constitute suicide under the legal system of the state. Physicians and patients who adhere to the law are protected from criminal prosecution, and participation cannot affect the status of a patient's health and life insurance policies.

What has been the experience under the Death with Dignity laws in the United States? One study,[3] which seems representative, reported that of 114 patients who inquired about a Death with Dignity program over about a three-year period, 39% chose not to pursue it and 26% initiated the process but did not complete it, either because they elected not to continue or they had died. The forty participants who remained, which was about a third (35%) of the initial number who inquired, received a prescription for a lethal dose of secobarbital. Of those forty who obtained a prescription, twenty-four (60%) chose to take the medication and died from it. The remaining sixteen patients did not take the medication and died of their illness. The most common reasons for participating in the program were interest in preserving autonomy (97%), inability to engage in enjoyable activities (89%), and loss of dignity (75%). The typical participant was male, white, and well educated.

What can we take from this? First, issues of autonomy, quality of life, and dignity seem to be most important for people who participate. Contrary to some concerns, experience in this study and others thus far indicates that people who are perceived as vulnerable do not seem to be disproportionately represented among those who choose to participate. Also, many people who inquire about the program choose not to participate and, more interesting, a high proportion of those who do participate and receive a prescription choose not to take the medication. This seems to be because patients value the control, the autonomy, the option to take the medication, even if they do not exercise the option. Patients also may change their minds about taking their own life.

WHAT IF I LIVE IN A STATE OR COUNTRY THAT DOES NOT PERMIT PHYSICIAN-ASSISTED DEATH?

This is the situation for most of us. Ideally, end-of-life matters can be dealt with by adequate pain control and other features of comfort care, which we talked about in Chapter 5. As death approaches, people often receive a drug such as morphine to ease their distress. Morphine calms, sedates, may obliterate consciousness in higher doses, and relieves the distress of labored breathing that often occurs before death. The latter effect on breathing also may hasten death by depressing the brain center that controls respiration. This is the so-called double effect of morphine, something that has been known for centuries and still plays an important part in end-of-life treatment. Moral, ethical, and legal questions associated with the double effect hinge on intent. If the intent of giving a terminal patient morphine is to relieve suffering, that is acceptable, compassionate care. If the intent is to kill the patient, that raises moral, ethical, and legal concerns.

A few dying people who want to take advantage of physician-assisted death laws might move, as did Brittany Maynard, to a state that permits it. Usually that is highly impractical. Moving is difficult for anyone and more so for someone who is terminally ill. People at the end of life generally want to remain with loved ones and in familiar surroundings. Also, establishing the requirements for residency may be complicated and take more time than they have to live.

VSED—VOLUNTARILY STOPPING EATING AND DRINKING

Another option for people to kill themselves, whether or not they live in a state or country that permits physician-assisted death, is to voluntarily stop eating and drinking. This is known as VSED.

John Rehm died June 23, 2014, a little more than a week after he made the decision to stop eating and drinking.[4] His decision to die came after a difficult conversation with his wife, Diane Rehm, author and former public radio show host, and his children and family physician. John was 83 years old and suffering from the debilitating effects of Parkinson's disease. Diane Rehm describes why he made his decision to die.

> John declared to Dr. Fried [his physician] that because Parkinson's disease had so affected him that he no longer had the use of his hands, arms or legs, because he could no longer stand, walk, eat, bathe, or in any way care for himself on his own, he was now ready to die. He said that he understood the disease was progressing, taking him further and further into incapacity, with no hope of improvement. Therefore, he wanted to end his life.

John had expected, now that he had made the decision to die, that Dr. Fried could help him die by prescribing the appropriate medication. But Dr. Fried explained that in the state of Maryland, where John lived, he was unable to acquiesce to John's request. John became angry and said, "I feel betrayed." He had been used to making his own decisions throughout his life and having them carried out. This ultimate decision was being thwarted. At this point Dr. Fried explained that the only alternative for John, if he wished to die, was to stop eating and drinking. That is what John did. The aides at the residential facility where he was living were instructed to stop bringing food, water, and medications, and he died nine days later.

VSED is growing in acceptance by terminally ill patients who, with support from families and caregivers, use it to end their lives. Complete cessation of eating and drinking requires great determination on the part of the terminally ill person and unswerving supportive assistance from caregivers, but it is remarkably effective. It causes death, mostly by dehydration, within one to two weeks. Of course, most people who choose VSED are ill and somewhat debilitated, so the effects of stopping all liquid and nutritional intake may be accelerated compared to a well person who does the same thing. Also, people who are approaching death typically have little appetite, which facilitates the lack of food intake during VSED. Stopping liquids makes people thirsty. Even sips of water prolong the dying process, so caregivers need to avoid giving water but should keep the person's mouth moistened to lessen the discomfort of thirst. Pain treatment continues as with any dying patient who has pain. The predictable pace of dying over one to two weeks, as compared to the immediate death that occurs after ingesting barbiturates in physician-assisted death, gives the dying person time to say goodbye and allows them to change their minds, until they lose consciousness.[5]

No laws specifically prohibit VSED and everyone has the right to refuse medical interventions. Whether eating and drinking are medical interventions is a matter of belief or perspective. Clearly, eating and drinking are an essential requirement to remaining alive and are characteristic of good health. But in a person who is dying, eating and drinking could be interpreted as a medical intervention. In some states, when a patient enters palliative care and requests cessation of all interventions, they or their surrogates must state specifically whether they want intravenous fluids and nutrition by feeding tube stopped; otherwise, IV fluids and a feeding tube will be continued.

Anyone, with sufficient resolve, can stop eating or drinking, whether they have a terminal illness or not. It does not require the assistance of a physician or health care professional or permission from the state. Because of this, people with non-malignant illnesses or who have dementia have used VSED to help them die. Dementia excludes a person from eligibility for assisted death in the states that permit it. But some people with Alzheimer's disease, with the help of loved ones and caregivers, who have previously expressed their desire not to live in the final stages of dementia, have used VSED to die. The application of VSED to demented patients and others who do not have full decision-making capacity is controversial, even if the person had expressed their wish not to live with advanced Alzheimer's disease or another form of dementia.

In Chapter 1, I pointed out the many ways that dying has changed over recent decades. I observe here that one thing has not changed: People always have had the option to stop eating and drinking. What has changed is now we have an official acronym for it!

SUICIDE IN NON-TERMINAL CONDITIONS

Some people, for whom physician-assisted death is not available legally or does not apply, or VSED does not seem right or doable, contemplate taking their own lives by other means.

The novelist Virginia Woolf, who seems to have suffered episodic severe depression, drowned herself March 28, 1941 by walking into a river near her home, her coat pockets filled with stones. The poignant letter she left her husband provides a glimpse into the mind of a person who has suffered extreme mental anguish and no longer can endure it. The letter begins, "Dearest, I feel certain I am going mad again. I feel we can't go through another of those terrible times. And I shan't recover this time. I begin to hear voices, and I can't concentrate. So I am doing what seems the best thing to do . . ."

Are mental illnesses that have been refractory to treatment, such as intractable depression or anorexia nervosa, which themselves may be a slow form of suicide over years, ever a justification for physician-assisted death? Existing Death with Dignity laws in the United States are careful to exclude anyone with mental illness from eligibility. This is not the case in The Netherlands, Belgium, and Switzerland, which allow assisted suicide for people with severe psychiatric disorders. The experience in The Netherlands, however, highlights some of the ambiguity and moral concern that arise when people with psychiatric disorders are permitted to kill themselves.[6] In that country, which requires that a person's psychiatric disorder be intractable and untreatable, even evaluating and deciding whether a patient suffers from an intractable and untreatable psychiatric illness may be imprecise. Also, although the most common diagnosis in The Netherlands is depression, it often coexists with other problems, such as substance abuse, dementia, chronic pain, and loneliness, which confound the diagnosis. Further, the observation that many depressed patients in

The Netherlands refused treatment for depression that could have helped them, choosing to die instead, raises additional concerns. I wonder whether easy access to state-sanctioned suicide may be an overreaching of the concept of patient autonomy, a person's right to choose.

For some people, who are not mentally ill and do not have a discrete terminal illness, experiencing the physical and mental deterioration and disability of aging is sufficient to convince them it is time to end their lives. Consider the story of this couple.

> Richard and Jo Hyse went to bed for the last time Nov. 8 (2009) in their Oswego (New York) house of 48 years. Their bags were packed for Florida the next day . . . Richard Hyse, 89, was an economics professor emeritus at the State University College at Oswego and Jo, 86, was a watercolor artist with a local gallery named in her honor. They were German Jews who survived World War II and immigrated to the United States after the communist takeover of East Berlin.[7]

Relatives had called the Hyses and received no response. Police were asked to investigate. They found the Hyses in their bedroom, both dead. Police said that Jo Hyse had swallowed eighteen OxyContin pills and she had been shot once in the head. Richard Hyse had taken twelve OxyContin pills along with a mixture of other drugs. Although both had experienced deterioration of their health in recent months, and Jo had become distressed by her forgetfulness and Richard had difficulty walking because of spine problems, neither was terminally ill. Family and acquaintances told police they were not surprised that the fiercely independent Hyses took their lives on their own terms. It is touching and curious that the Hyses packed their bags for the trip to Florida before killing themselves. What does that mean? Of course, all we can do is speculate.

Others, who do not necessarily have a terminal illness but have had enough of life and who live in a country, or can travel to one, where assisted suicide is available, effectively on request, may choose that option to kill themselves. The dual suicides of Sir Edward Downes, distinguished British orchestra conductor, and his wife were public, dramatic examples.[8] They flew to Switzerland in July 2009 where they both drank a lethal cocktail of barbiturates at an assisted-suicide clinic. Friends of the Downses said that Sir Edward was not known to have a terminal illness, but he had declared that he wanted to die with his wife of over fifty years, who had been ill.

Although still uncommon, such voluntary ending of one's life, when one is not terminally ill, seems more prevalent. Perhaps because people are living longer, some choose not to tolerate the consequent deterioration and debilitation of aging, and they take the opportunity to end their lives peacefully and non-traumatically, if it is available. Some of the appeal of such a death may be that it can be planned and even orchestrated to occur in the presence of loved ones who will remember you as you want to be remembered, not as someone who has deteriorated bit by bit and is, at last, not the person you were. One prominent bioethicist has gone a step further. Ezekiel Emanuel, when he was age 57, declared that he hoped to die at 75.[9] He argued that living too long

> . . . renders many of us, if not disabled, then faltering and declining, a state that may not be worse than death but is nonetheless deprived. It robs us of our creativity and ability to contribute to work, society, the world. It transforms how people experience us, relate to us, and, most important, remember us. We are no longer remembered as vibrant and engaged but as feeble, ineffectual, even pathetic.

Advocates for Death with Dignity laws might use these accounts as evidence that such laws should be available everywhere or even expanded to include people whose expected death is longer than six months. Opponents might say that these are examples of unjustified suicide, perhaps even murder, or inappropriate use of existing laws.

These experiences raise additional questions. What are the limits of autonomy, of personal choice and freedom? Should society not only permit but provide the means for someone to kill herself almost at will? Of course, anyone can kill herself, but is it right that one's society condones it?

You undoubtedly have your own opinions about physician-assisted death and other methods of terminating one's life under the circumstances we have discussed. Perhaps those views will be reinforced or will change as you become more familiar with end-of-life matters through your own experiences with loved ones, friends, or yourself.

Regardless of our views, the experiences of the Hyses and the Downeses evoke the notions we all as individuals hold about quality of life and what life means to us that we talked about in Chapter 2. We live longer now than our parents and grandparents, thanks to the advances in public health and medical care that we talked about in Chapter 1, but is more life better? It depends on the circumstances, doesn't it? Having more control over our death, whether by making our wishes known (Chapter 3), choosing comfort care (Chapter 5), or actually taking our own life, may allow us to have more control over the parts at the end of life that are important to us. If dying at home, in the company of loved ones and friends is important, perhaps we can do that or approximate it by having more control over the other circumstances of our death. And, how we deal with our death, even to the extent of causing it ourselves, contributes to the story that each of us creates about our own life, throughout our life, until the end. Let's try to understand more about our own life story in the next chapter.

Chapter 7
FINISHING OUR STORY

The web of our life is of a mingled yarn, good and ill together.
      —William Shakespeare, *All's Well That Ends Well*

Each of us creates a story of our life. We begin to gather material for the story in infancy and childhood. By adolescence the narrative starts to take form and we compose it, modify it, rearrange it, and interpret it for the rest of our lives, telling it to ourselves as we put our actions and our experiences in context, and telling it to others each time we share who we are and where we've been and what we've done. To get to know someone, to make a connection with another person—that act that is so central to human life and relationships—is to tell our story and to hear and learn another person's.

Psychologist Dan McAdams puts it this way: "A life story is a personal myth that an individual begins working on in late adolescence and young adulthood in order to provide his or her life with unity or purpose . . . " He defines that personal myth as ". . . a special kind of story that each of us naturally constructs to bring together the different parts of ourselves and our lives into a purposeful and convincing whole. Like all stories, the personal myth has a beginning, a middle, and end, defined according to the development of plot and character."[1]

Our life story can be fulfilling, heroic, scary, tragic, ironic, comic, or a mix of several themes. It is a story that develops around a framework of facts and experiences, but it is not so much about facts as it is about meanings; it is highly interpretive. It is truthful in the sense that all myths represent certain essential truths. The truths may be more about how we felt about something when it was happening or how we feel about it now, rather than any objective description of an event or experience. The story has many chapters and is susceptible to editing. "We all, as we grow old, meddle with the storyline of our lives, edit stuff out, re-cast the darker passages in a kindlier light," writes spy genre author David Cornwell.[2]

As we get older, we may think more about the legacy we will leave when we die. In the first chapter, I talked about the desire to delay the aging process, to extend life and delay death, perhaps to recapture our youth, or even to achieve immortality. Our legacy is a form of immortality. How will others remember us? The story we have created, for ourselves and for others, is an essential part of our legacy, how we will be remembered. McAdams writes, "All good stories require a satisfying ending. As we move into and through our middle-adult years, we become increasingly preoccupied with our own myth's denouement. Few of us are eager to die. Mature identity requires that we leave a legacy that will, in some sense, survive us." Our story is a gift to the next generation. "We recast and revise our own life stories so that the past is seen as giving birth to the present and the future, and so that beginning, middle, and end make sense in terms of each other. A legacy of the self is generated and offered up to others . . ."[1] We work on our story until we die.

THE LAST CHAPTER

The end of life is an important chapter of our story. It is an opportunity to conclude the story in a way that satisfies us, and that may be acceptable to others in our lives, and to contribute to the meaning with which we already have imbued the story. It also is the last chance, as the author and editor of our own story, to make revisions. I'm not saying that you can change or undo something you did years ago. I am saying that there may be opportunities for you to put experiences into a renewed context and derive a different meaning from them. After all, you are the author of your own story and, although you cannot change facts or experiences, you might be able to modify what some of them mean to you or see them in a new light.

As life unfolds and more of life is behind than in front, there is more for us to review and put in its proper place. Our understandings of life and of our own story may mature. Perhaps this is a piece of what is called wisdom. But are we completely satisfied with the story? Are there any loose ends, incomplete subplots, regrets, mistakes, or misunderstandings that should be redressed? Is this a time to remedy old grudges, to reconcile? Should we reconnect with old friends, revisit places that have had meaning for us, and put a little more energy into our current relationships? Do we wish to be remembered in a little different way?

If we want to change our narrative late in life, can we actually do it? And how do we do it? As the saying goes, Can a leopard change its spots? Perhaps. Or are we like some authors who claim they have little control over their stories, that what they write seems to come almost unbidden from some source deep within the repository of their thoughts and experience? And thus the end of life will unfold in some inevitable, automatic fashion, unaffected by any conscious intervention to modify the story line. I am an optimist and believe we can change within imperfect parameters of character and will.

I do not have the hubris to tell you how you should think and behave during the end of your life. One's fundamental values and character, and attitudes and behaviors, are not likely to change substantially. Whatever you do at the end of your life is likely to be consistent with whatever has gone on before. But I do have some suggestions about what you should consider in preparing for the end of life and living it when you get there, that may give you better say over the final chapter and make it more meaningful and satisfying for you and the people you care about.

SUGGESTIONS TO PREPARE FOR AND MANAGE THE END OF LIFE AND MAKE IT MORE FULFILLING

- At any time of your life, but certainly in your mature and later years, consider what could happen to you under different health and social circumstances. Discuss these with another person, perhaps your spouse or partner, or a close relative or a friend. If you have a chronic disorder, say, diabetes, heart trouble, kidney disease, or a neurological condition, what futures do people with those conditions often have? Can you anticipate the kinds of decisions you might have to make? If you are healthy, can you envision a time when you are not healthy and how would you deal with that? Perhaps you know someone, a parent, a relative, or a friend, who has been in a situation that has made you more aware of possibilities you might face someday. What about those situations do you think you could control? If you lost your cognitive ability or otherwise could not speak for yourself, how could you prepare for that? Would you want to make your wishes known in advance? What would be your wishes regarding specific treatments if you were in a futile medical situation? Are there circumstances in which you would want a Do Not Resuscitate or Do Not Intubate order written for you?

- Reflect on the importance of quality of life to you. Quality-of-life questions may arise at any time during our life story, from beginning to end, but they are characteristic features of the last chapter. What does quality of life mean to you? What gives your life meaning? Are there aspects of the quality of your life that are more important than others? Would severe restriction or loss of your quality of life guide some end-of-life decisions for you? Or is what people conventionally call quality of life of less importance to you than the sustaining of biological life, meaning, in end-of-life dramas, "doing everything" to be kept alive is what you wish?

- Select a health care proxy (HCP) agent. In light of what we talked about in Chapter 3, your HCP agent should be someone you trust who understands your wishes, after conversations with you, and who can represent your wishes, not their own, unless they happen to coincide with yours. And choose someone who, although they may love you, can be dispassionate enough to make good decisions for you. Then execute an HCP document, or a living will, keep the original for yourself, and give copies to your HCP agent, your main physician, and anyone else you think should have one.

- Decide who else needs to be included in your end-of-life planning. Do you need to share your thoughts with your children and other relatives and friends?

- If where you will die is important to you, specify that to your HCP agent and other loved ones, so your wishes regarding this can be respected if possible.

- Bear in mind that some of the characters who populated the earlier chapters of your story are likely to reappear in the last chapter. What are the implications of that to you?

- Try to pay up your emotional debts. Is there someone to whom you need to apologize or explain an earlier behavior? This seems good advice at any time of life.
- On the nostalgia scale, I am at the high end. If you are up there, too, I suggest that you reinforce memories and simultaneously prepare for the end of life by revisiting places that have meaning to you, reconnecting with friends and others, and reliving experiences, such as re-reading books, watching special movies, and listening to favorite music.

We write the final chapter of our story as certainly as we write all the preceding chapters, with the caveat that some of the authorship may have to be shared with others. Leave as little as you can to your proxy authors, and what you must leave to them, try to make sure it is written as you would have written it yourself.

REFERENCES

CHAPTER 1

1. "Where Do Americans Die?" Stanford School of Medicine, Palliative Care. https://palliative.stanford.edu/home-hospice-home-care-of-the-dying-patient/where-do-americans-die/.

2. "10 FAQs: Medicare's Role in End-of-Life Care," The Henry J. Kaiser Family Foundation, November 2015.

3. "Deaths: Final Data for 2010," Centers for Disease Control and Prevention, National Vital Statistics Report, Table 3, 2013;61(4). http://www.cdc.gov/nchs/data/nvsr/nvsr61/nvsr61_04.pdf.

4. Gerald F. Riley, James D. Lubitz, "Long-Term Trends in Medicare Payments in the Last Year of Life," *Health Services Research* 2010;45(2):565–76.

5. Max Ehrenfreund, "The Stunning—and Expanding—Gap in Life Expectancy Between the Rich and the Poor," *Washington Post*, September 18, 2015.

6. Raj Chetty, Michael Stepner, Sarah Abraham, Shelby Lin, Benjamin Scuderi, Nicholas Turner, Augustin Bergeron, David Cutler, "The Association Between Income and Life Expectancy in the United States, 2001–2014," *Journal of the American Medical Association* 2016;315(16):1750–66.

7. Gina Kolata, "Death Rates Rising for Middle-Aged White Americans, Study Finds," *New York Times*, November 2, 2015.

8. "Country Comparison: Life Expectancy at Birth," The World Factbook, Central Intelligence Agency. https://www.cia.gov/library/publications/the-world-factbook/rankorder/2102rank.html.

9. Tad Friend, "Silicon Valley's Quest to Live Forever. Can Billions of Dollars' Worth of High-Tech Research Succeed in Making Death Optional?" *The New Yorker*, April 3, 2017.

10. "Scientists Identify New Molecular Pathway That Controls Aging," *Sci-News*, October 16, 2017.

11. "The Public and Genetic Editing, Testing, and Therapy," *STAT. Harvard School of Public Health*, January 2016. https://cdn1.sph.harvard.edu/wp-content/uploads/sites/94/2016/01/STAT-Harvard-Poll-Jan-2016-Genetic-Technology.pdf.

12. "Living to 120 and Beyond: Americans' Views on Aging, Medical Advances and Radical Life Extension," Pew Research Center, August 6, 2013.

http://www.pewforum.org/2013/08/06/living-to-120-and-beyond-americans-views-on-aging-medical-advances-and-radical-life-extension/.

13. JF Dasta, TP McLaughlin, SH Mody, CT Piech, "Daily Cost of an Intensive Care Unit Day: The Contribution of Mechanical Ventilation," *Critical Care Medicine* 2005 June;33(6):1266–71.

14. "Patient Pricing Information," University Hospitals of Cleveland, January 2, 2018. http://www.uhhospitals.org/rainbow/patients-and-visitors/billing-insurance-and-medical-records/patient-pricing-information.

CHAPTER 2

1. Anna Reisman, "Gifts," *New England Journal of Medicine* 2016;374:208–209.

CHAPTER 3

1. Erin S. DeMartino, David M. Dudzinski, Cavan K. Doyle, Beau P. Sperry, Sarah E. Gregory, Mark Siegler, Daniel P. Sulmasy, Paul S. Mueller, Daniel K. Kramer, "Who Decides When a Patient Can't? Statutes on Alternate Decision Makers," *New England Journal of Medicine* 2017;376:1478–82.

CHAPTER 5

1. This and other names in this account are fictitious.

2. Pedro Gozalo, Michael Plotzke, Vincent Mor, Susan C. Miller, Joan M. Teno, "Changes in Medicare Costs with the Growth of Hospice Care in Nursing Homes," *New England Journal of Medicine* 2015;372:1823–31.

3. Amy S. Kelley, R. Sean Morrison, "Palliative Care for the Seriously Ill," *New England Journal of Medicine* 2015;373:747–55.

4. Craig D. Blinderman, J. Andrew Billings, "Comfort Care for Patients Dying in the Hospital," *New England Journal of Medicine* 2015;373:2549–61.

CHAPTER 6

1. Lindsey Bever, "Brittany Maynard, as promised, ends her life at 29," *Washington Post*, November 2, 2014.

2. "Death with Dignity Act Requirements," State of Oregon, https://public.health.oregon.gov/ProviderPartnerResources/EvaluationResearch/DeathwithDignityAct/Documents/requirements.pdf.

3. Elizabeth Trice Loggers, Helene Starks, Moreen Shannon-Dudley, Anthony L. Back, Frederick R. Applebaum, F. Marc Stewart, "Implementing a Death with Dignity Program at a Comprehensive Cancer Center," *New England Journal of Medicine* 2013;368:1417–24.

4. Diane Rehm, *On My Own*. New York: Alfred A. Knopf, 2016.

5. Paula Span, "The VSED Exit: A Way to Speed Up Dying, Without Asking Permission," *New York Times*, October 21, 2016.

6. Benedict Carey, "Assisted Suicide Study Questions Its Use for Mentally Ill," *New York Times*, February 10, 2016.

7. Douglass Dowty, "For Oswego Couple, Home Was Where Their Hearts Were," *Syracuse, NY Post-Standard*, April 18, 2010.
8. John F. Burns, "With Help, Conductor and Wife Ended Lives," *New York Times*, July 15, 2009.
9. Ezekiel J. Emanuel, "Why I Hope to Die at 75," *The Atlantic*, October 2014.

CHAPTER 7
1. Dan P. McAdams, *The Stories We Live By. Personal Myths and the Making of the Self.* New York: Guilford Press, 1993.
2. Adam Sisman, *John le Carre. The Biography.* New York: HarperCollins, 2015.

INDEX